D0791093

Older Mothers

Conception, pregnancy and birth after 35

Julia Berryman, Karen Thorpe and Kate Windridge

Pandora
An Imprint of Rivers Oram Press

For our children –
Tom, Amy, Grace and Emily

Pandora
An imprint of Rivers Oram Press
144 Hemingford Road
London N1 1DE

Published by Pandora 1995
Reprinted 1998

© Julia Berryman, Karen Thorpe and Kate Windridge 1995

Julia Berryman, Karen Thorpe and Kate Windridge assert the moral
right to be identified as the authors of this work

A catalogue record for this book
is available from the British Library

ISBN 0 865358 410 1 (pb)

Printed and bound by
Caledonian International, Bishopbriggs, Scotland

All rights reserved. No part of this publication may be reproduced,
stored in a retrieval system, or transmitted, in any form or by any
means, electronic, mechanical, photocopying, recording or
otherwise, without the prior permission of the publisher.

Contents

Start reading this book at whichever point – chapter, subheading or page – interests you most. Each chapter is relatively self-contained to enable you to read in this way. References are made to other chapters as appropriate.

Acknowledgements

There are many, many people who have helped us in the course of our work preparing this book and we should like to thank all of them. The book would not have been possible without them.

First and foremost we should like to thank the women who have taken part, and are continuing to take part, in our various studies of later motherhood. All three of us have researched this topic over many years and in that time many hundreds, and sometimes thousands, of women have been interviewed, filled in questionnaires and answered questions on all aspects of motherhood. We should like to thank all those who took part in the British research: the British study of 40-plus mothers, the Leicester Motherhood Project, the Egg Donation Project, and the Avon Longitudinal Study of Pregnancy and Childhood (the Children of the Nineties study). Thanks also to the participants in the Australian Timing of Motherhood study and the Greek preliminary study for the European Longitudinal Study of Pregnancy and Childhood. Funding for these projects has been from a variety of sources and we should particularly like to thank Nestlé UK Ltd for their support of our Leicester research and the Leicester University Research Board for their pump-priming grant.

There are many individuals to whom we owe so much; for statistical advice, John Beckett and Bill Williamson in Leicester, Rosemary Greenwood in Bristol, and Richard Startup in Swansea; for help with analysis of data, Rosemary Greenwood in

Bristol and Sylvia West in Leicester; for data preparation, Sue Williams in Leicester and the dedicated staff of ALSPAC in Bristol. Special thanks go to Jean Golding, director of ALSPAC, for her kind permission to report results from this study. In Brisbane, Australia, thanks to the computing staff at the University of Queensland, department of Psychology, and to Jana Cinnamon who worked with Karen Thorpe on the Australian Timing of Motherhood study. We are also very grateful to Steve Rawlinson for help with literature searches, Sue Smith who has been a source of much advice on population statistics, and Linda Huig for locating and photocopying endless articles, all at Leicester University Library, and thanks also to Pam Gibson at Leicester University computer centre who rescued a previously unreadable file containing two vital chapters of the final manuscript!

John MacVicar, Professor of Obstetrics and Gynaecology at Leicester University, was a major source of advice, encouragement and support at the start of our Leicester research, which could not have been carried out without the personal involvement of many staff at Leicester Royal Infirmary including Janet Holland, Margaret Hopkins, Maureen Keating, Julia Savage, Linda Stockwell and all those who work with them. Thank you.

Very special thanks are due to Steph Kneller who has provided support far beyond the ready deployment of her considerable word-processing skills. We thank her for shouldering much of the last minute pressure in preparing the manuscript, for weekend dog-sitting whilst we wrote, and for generally keeping up our spirits – we could not have managed without her.

There are some important friends and relations whom we should like to acknowledge here: all have given us 'food for thought', whether through describing their own feelings about parenting or through allowing us to try out ideas on them. They are Rob Allen, Penny Allerton, Ruby and Eric Berryman, Ros. Castell, Trudy Goodenough, Rosemary Greenwood, Pam Hardman, Gillie Harries, Alison Pike, Bobbie Stormont, Keith Stevenson, Maggie Stevenson-Leggett, Sophie Wellstood, Vivienne Williams and Anne Windridge. Karen would particularly like to thank Janvrin Edbrooke, and also the staff of the Tin

Drum Nursery, Bristol – the latter for taking extra care of Emily while Karen was writing.

On a more personal note we turn to our immediate families. Thanking them adequately is difficult, as they have put up with more than could reasonably be expected while we immersed ourselves in the work. Our respective husbands and children have somehow continued to love and support us throughout. The latter have been motherless, or perhaps we should say mother-free, for longer periods than we would have liked, the former have taken over more than their share of domestic chores and child-care and still been patient and interested enough to find time to read endless drafts of chapters while they were 'in preparation', and to comment on them from their own perspectives . . . so thank you to Philip and Tom Drew, Emily and Nick Sawyer, and Grace, Amy and Paul Windridge. Much as we have enjoyed writing this book there have been many times when we have sorely missed your company. However, without you this book would never even have been conceived.

Permissions

Table 2.1 Fertility Ratio of the Hutterites and Selected Populations. Source Eaton and Mayer, 1953. Eaton, J.W. and Mayer, A.J. (1953). The social biology of very high fertility among the Hutterites: The demography of a unique population. *Human Biology*, 25(3), 206–264. Reprinted by permission of the author Joseph Eaton. Wayne State University Press now control rights to material published in *Human Biology* and these publishers indicate that this material is in the public domain and permission from the publisher is not required.

Table 2.2 Number of Children Still Possible per Woman After Any Given Age by Five Year Age Groups, for the Ethnic Hutterite Women Living in December 31 1950. Source Eaton and Mayer, 1953. Eaton, J.W. & Mayer, A.J. (1953). The social biology of very high fertility among the Hutterites: The demography of a unique population. *Human Biology*, 25(3), 206–264. Reprinted by permission, as for Table 2.1 above.

Table 2.3 The Percentage of Live Births in England and Wales, by Maternal Age, Born to Women in 1992. Adapted from Birth Statistics, 1992. Birth Statistics, 1992 (1994). Review of the Registrar General on births and patterns of family building in England and Wales. Series FM1 no. 21. London: HMSO. Reprinted by permission of HMSO.

Table 4.1 Natural Fertility: The Average of Age-specific Fertility Rates for 13 Populations Not Practising Birth Control. Source Henry's data 1961. Henry, L. (1961). Some data on natural fertility. *Eugenics Quarterly*. 8, 81–91. Reprinted by permission of the Editor of Social Biology who controls copyright of this material.

Table 4.2 Age-specific Percentages of Sterility in Married Women. Source Henry's data, 1961. Henry L. (1961). Some data on natural fertility. *Eugenics Quarterly*. 8, 81–91. Reprinted by permission, as for Table 4.1 above.

Table 4.3 The Success of AID by Age of Women. Source Schwartz and Mayaux, 1982. Schwartz, D. & Mayaux, M.J. (1982). Female fecundity as a function of age. *New England Journal of Medicine*, 306(7) 404–406. Reprinted by permission of the publishers of the New England Journal of Medicine and the authors.

Table 4.5 Range of Incidence of Miscarriage by Maternal Age. Source Hansen, 1986. Hansen, J. (1986). Older maternal age and pregnancy outcome: a review of the literature. *Obstetrical & Gynecological Survey*, 41(11), 726–34. Reprinted by permission of the author and publisher/copyright holder Williams & Wilkins.

Table 4.6 Miscarriage Rate in Women Undergoing Artificial Insemination. Source Virro and Shewchek, 1984. Virro, M.R. & Shewchuk, A.B. (1984). Pregnancy outcome in 242 conceptions after artificial insemination and donor sperm and effects of maternal age on the prognosis for successful pregnancy. *American Journal of Obstetrics and Gynecology*, 148, 518–524.

Table 5.1 Age of mothers and risk of Down's syndrome (trisomy 21), Edward's syndrome (trisomy 18), Patau's Syndrome (trisomy 13) and sex chromosome abnormalities (XXY or XXX) in the child. Sources: (1) Donnai, D (1988) Genetic Risk in D.K. James and G.M. Stirrat (1988) *Pregnancy and Risk*. John Wiley and Sons. (2) James, D.K. (1988) Risk at Booking in D.K. James and G.M. Stirrat (1988). *Pregnancy and Risk*. John Wiley and Sons. Reprinted by permission of the editors: D.K. James and G.M. Stirrat.

Table 9.1 Proportion of women with pre-school children who are in paid employment in selected countries. Source: Brannen, J. and Moss, P. (1988) *New Mothers at Work*, London: Unwin

Introduction

The need for a book on conception, pregnancy and birth after 35 seemed very clear to us. We have all been immersed in researching the topic of maternal age and its impact on motherhood: the psychological aspects as well as the medical aspects of pregnancy, birth, and afterwards. There are a number of books available on later motherhood – some are 'how to' books that are designed for women themselves considering later motherhood, and others are accounts of women's experiences showing, through anecdotes, what it is like – the good and the bad points. All these sources have an important role in informing would-be mothers but until now books have not attempted to cover comprehensively the research exploring the impact of a mother's age on her experience of motherhood.

Our book is designed to present the available evidence and to discover whether there are real differences between older and younger mothers. Anecdotal accounts always have an important place in illustrating how individuals feel but they can give, even unintentionally, a distorted view of what the experience is like for the majority of people in a given group. Our aim is to place each individual account or research study into the whole context of women who are 35-plus mothers: to take the wider view. We have drawn on our own broad research experience – between us we have been involved in studies in Britain, Greece, and Australia – and we have looked at all the available international research that has thrown light on motherhood after 35; in particular we have drawn on several in-depth studies carried out in Britain, Australia and the United States including our own research. Later motherhood is nothing new but the reasons for it today, in the 1990s, are quite different from those that applied even a few decades ago. Women's patterns of paid working have changed dramatically, as has family life. Very few families are just mum, dad and two children – today there are many single parent families, families including step-children, and parents who are remarried or in new partnerships; there are extended families with grandparents and other relatives within the home, and there are families made up of lesbian or gay partners and their children. The variety in family life is enormous.

This book takes a magnifying glass to 'older' mothers – and we have defined such women as those who have a baby on or after their thirty-fifth birthday: for simplicity's sake we call them 35-plus mothers. We have looked at the kinds of women who start or add to their families at this stage in life and describe them in all their variety. The book contains the objective facts and the statistics – such as 'Who has babies after 35?' in Chapter 2, and the subjective experiences in other chapters such as Chapter 6, which describes what pregnancy is like after 35. We have made the book a mix of the objective evidence on the topics under discussion, set beside the psychological perspective: the experiences that women have as they go through pregnancy, birth and motherhood.

This book is aimed at all those with an interest in, or a concern for, 35-plus mothers. We hope that all health professionals will find it a fund of information on a group of women whose numbers are increasing every year. We also hope that women contemplating motherhood themselves will find this an invaluable source of information. 35-plus mothers are the fastest growing group of mothers in many developed countries such as Britain, America and Australia. We need to know more about them and their experiences. This book seeks to provide a rich source of information based on all the evidence currently available. We hope you enjoy reading it as much as we enjoyed writing it.

Julia Berryman, Karen Thorpe & Kate Windridge
February 1995

Julia C. Berryman B.Sc., Ph.D., A.F.B.P.s.S., C.Psychol., is a Senior Lecturer in Psychology at the University of Leicester. She completed her first degree at the University of Aberdeen and her Ph.D. at Leicester University. She has researched and published widely on developmental psychology, sex and gender, parenthood and parenting. She set up the Parenthood Research Group at Leicester University and has investigated a variety of aspects of parenthood and motherhood and she currently directs the Leicester Motherhood Project, which is a longitudinal study of women of all ages, designed to highlight the effects of age and parity on women's experience of motherhood. The idea for this book on older mothers arose out of her research studies – the British study of 40-plus mothers and the Leicester Motherhood Project – both of which were carried out with her Research Associate, Dr Kate Windridge. Julia Berryman is the mother of a young son, Tom, born when she was 41 years old.

Karen Thorpe B.Ed., M.A., Ph.D., is a Research Fellow at the University of Bristol, Department of Child Health. She completed her first degree in Australia and subsequently studied Child Psychology at the University of London Institute of Education and the University of Bristol where she obtained her Ph.D. She has published papers on a wide range of subjects in the field of child development and parenthood. For the past five years she has worked on a study of 15,000 mothers, their partners, and children – the Avon Longitudinal Study of Pregnancy and Childhood. In 1992 she conducted a study of the timing of motherhood at the University of Queensland, Australia and she is currently working on a study of families with twins in a joint project with the MRC Unit of the Institute of Psychiatry in London. In 1994, during the writing of this book, at the age of 33, she became the proud mother of a daughter, Emily Florence.

Kate Windridge B.Sc., P.G.Cert.Ed., Ph.D., is a Research Associate with the Parenthood Research Group at Leicester University. She obtained her B.Sc. in Psychology, Music and Philosophy at Leicester University and spent some time as an aspiring rock musician before studying for a post-graduate teaching qualification, followed by a Ph.D. in Developmental Psychology. Since then she has spent over ten years teaching psychology and carrying out research in university and hospital settings, and she has published widely. Currently she is working on the Leicester Motherhood Project and is the mother of two daughters, Grace and Amy, both born when she was over the age of 30.

৯ 1 ৯

Motherhood after 35:
Case Histories

What kinds of women have babies after 35? Are they career women fitting a child into a busy professional life, women having babies within second marriages, women adjusting to unexpected arrivals or single women deciding to go it alone? The most striking aspect of our research into this issue has been that it is impossible to pigeon-hole such women. Each woman is unique so that her own story involves a variety of life events which make her experiences unlike all others. To begin our explorations we have chosen a selection of personal accounts by real women who have had babies after 35 to give a sample of the wide range of experiences that can lead to a later baby. We have changed some details in order to preserve anonymity in this chapter and throughout the book, but the accounts that follow remain true to the spirit of each woman's experiences. We have chosen some dramatic stories and some more straightforward ones; we have also included women who are trying to decide whether or not to become mothers after 35, who describe their thoughts and feelings during the decision-making process. This chapter highlights, through the following case histories, many of the issues which are to be discussed in the rest of the book.

ॐ
Unplanned pregnancies:
joy versus devastation

Joy . . .

MAUREEN: 41, A FRESH BEGINNING

Maureen had not planned her pregnancy. She was not part of a couple in the conventional sense and she had very little contact with her baby's father after conception. Her answers to our questions were among the most positive of all those we received. She reported very low levels of depression, few worries, few health problems and so on.

When Maureen had first got married she had assumed that she and her husband would have children within a few years, but *'material things and money became more important.'* Despite thinking very seriously about children when she was 30, Maureen did not try to get pregnant because her husband still did not want children. Then, all in the same year, her mother died, she and her husband separated . . . and she became pregnant, at the age of 41. She was unsure who had fathered the baby as she had met a new boyfriend while on holiday abroad and had not used contraception as she thought she was (but *'half hoped'* she was not) too old to conceive.

The doctors who saw her were convinced that the baby was her ex-husband's.

> *My husband's had a vasectomy . . . and by my dates my boyfriend must be the father, but when I had the scan it suggested my ex was the father. My GP said he'd never doubted that it was my husband's anyway.*

Maureen was not convinced and even when the baby was one she was still referring to her boyfriend as the 'real' father.

When she told her ex-husband that she was pregnant he was not happy. Her boyfriend, however, was delighted and she enjoyed his support although they were in contact only by phone, and had no long term plans to 'settle down' together.

How did other people react?

> *My mother-in-law says I'm irresponsible at my age, in my situation
> . . . I should have had more sense; but I expected it from her, I know her
> moral attitude and it's not particularly upset me . . . My brother has
> amazed me. We've never been close till now; it's brought us lots closer.*
>
> *I expected to be offered a termination because of my age. My GP
> asked how I felt. I didn't mind him saying that. I said, if you mean do I
> want a termination, no I don't. The staff at the hospital all made a
> special effort to discuss things because of my age.*

Overall Maureen was quite happy at the prospect of being a
single parent. She felt in fact that she was a lot happier and a lot
more fortunate than other pregnant women.

> *I've got a high paid job, a home which will be mine after the divorce, a
> very supportive family . . . and I'm lucky to be having a baby at my
> age.*

ELAINE: 37, UNEXPLAINED INFERTILITY

Like Maureen, Elaine was delighted at the prospect of having an
'unplanned' baby. She was 37 and had been married for 11 years.
Her husband was four years older. They had started trying for a
baby ten years before our interview, when Elaine had given up the
pill. After two years and no success she had had infertility investigations which included a laparoscopy after which she'd been
described as '99 per cent fertile'.

> *I felt very unhappy after the treatment* [laparoscopy] *and decided not
> to continue. I felt that I was not a 'normal' woman and seeing women
> with babies upset me. My husband did not really understand how I was
> feeling and we had relationship problems for a while after.*
>
> *When moving to this area I consulted my new doctor who was very
> understanding. Two years later we decided to go private. We were*

treated very well and realized what a common problem it was. However, after two stressful sessions of treatment we decided to let nature take its course. If it wasn't meant, that was OK. I think I had given up hope. All the people we saw during the treatment could find no problems physically with either of us.

Two years after abandoning any form of treatment Elaine became pregnant and at our interview she was well into her pregnancy at 19 weeks. The pregnancy was an unexpected joy because Elaine and her husband had felt that, *'though we'd like children, we'd accepted our life as it was.'* She described how her view of her future had, as a matter of course, included having a child one day. She came from a big family and the prospect of no children was a sad one.

Of the unexpected pregnancy she said she and her husband were:

Very happy at the moment. It's something we've wanted for years. We are both excited about having a child and feel our lifestyle and age is an advantage as we are both professional people who have worked hard, travelled and have many good friends and a supportive family.

Her baby was healthy and the family have settled down happily together. Elaine went back to work part-time when the baby was three months old, and feels overall that, although she might have been physically stronger when she was younger, her age was to her advantage:

I feel I've done lots of things; had full-time exciting jobs, so I'm not desperate to do those things now. She's come at the right time really: she's not hindered me. So many women get frustrated that they've not had a career.

Most of the women I mix with are eight to ten years younger, but it doesn't make any difference.

. . . and devastation

HELENA: 35, NEWLY ALONE, UNEXPECTED PREGNANCY

Helena's story stood out among all the others we encountered because of the number of misfortunes she faced. She had been married in her late teens but she and her husband had parted several years previously. She had continued to pursue her career as a lecturer in further education, and met a second partner.

I lived with someone else. I left him because neither of us had got over our marriages. Then I became pregnant. He went berserk when I told him. In his defence this had happened to him before. He offered to pay for a termination because he said he was not prepared to stand by me, but I've decided to keep the baby and he is now [mid-pregnancy] *sort of prepared to be involved. Now he says he really wants children but that he doesn't want one with me if the relationship isn't working . . . I put* [his] *hand on my tummy and he pulled away.*

How did *she* feel about babies?

I used to feel embarrassed when I saw small babies because they always cried when I held them. I was intensely jealous of a friend who was pregnant but also felt pressured by women who talked as if motherhood was the 'be-all and end-all'. I couldn't talk about babies all the time. I've a horror of it; the change in some of my friends who've had children is frightening, but I suppose it's like buying a new washing machine: if you meet someone else who's bought the same one you talk about it.

And how does she feel, at mid-pregnancy, about her situation?

How do I feel now? That's difficult to answer. Not maternal: it feels odd to have someone else inside me. It is miraculous, though, I'm glad to be living through it. When I had a car accident recently it was the baby I was worried about, also when I had my operation [emergency surgery during pregnancy] *. . . I did feel intense joy when I discovered I was pregnant . . . The thought of living alone but with a child* *holds out a lot more hope than living alone. I couldn't live with myself if I had a termination. My mother was adamant that I shouldn't have it but she's supporting me nevertheless.*

Pregnancy continued to be difficult. After the birth she looked back:

I was fine till about 30 weeks and then I felt [as if] I couldn't grow any more, I couldn't stretch. I felt ugly, grotesque . . . I started to hate myself. Then there were major, major, major hassles with the father. He said he wanted to be part of the labour if I allowed it, having not contacted me for weeks and weeks, and never visiting me all the time I was in hospital . . . He also came to antenatal classes with me. That was awful because it was all about couples and he made it very clear he didn't want anything to do with me.

Her ex-partner did attend the labour and was present at the birth.

I was scared that she wasn't going to be OK. Scared of seeing her. I did not want a boy but wouldn't admit it, not even to myself. I couldn't identify with bringing up a boy on my own. I cried my eyes out because she was a girl. Giving birth . . . was heart-rending because I knew the father wouldn't be there afterwards.

After the birth, life was still difficult. The baby *'screamed incessantly, I ached in every limb I was so tired, I cried and cried.'* The GP was concerned about the baby's health and

referred her to a paediatrician, who said she was just a wilful baby and I had to leave her crying or she'd have behavioural problems later. I tried leaving her the next day but by the time she'd screamed for three hours my nerves were shattered. I've never left her to cry since. She still screams [at five months] but I nurse her . . . I feel as if she's in a black hole, maybe in pain.

Then came a turning point in her feelings for the baby's father.

I suppose he's done me a good turn by making me loathe him. We had a massive row . . . he came and took her out without my permission and without telling me . . . then he turned it back on me saying he was doing me a favour, which is what he always does. I hit him and he walloped me back and told me he'd ring Social Services and say I was unfit to be a mother. I contacted the health visitor to see where I stood and she reassured me totally. My GP was superb, she said she'd support me 100 per cent.

What other support had she had?

The health visitor and my mum are both marvellous. It was the health visitor who actually cracked me. I was putting on a brave face and she pressed me, and I burst into tears and told her everything. I'm on antidepressants now and they've really helped.

At one year she said that the baby was still very insecure and had health problems.

It's been a struggle all the way through. I've caught everything she's had . . . my health and her health have been major issues. I'm still taking antidepressants . . . But she's given me great confidence. It makes me step out and approach others because it does her good. It's made me realize I'm a fighter and I don't give up easily. She's been a challenge, but a great pleasure.

Life is still a matter of survival from day to day but much of the stress has lifted . . . She is still a highly strung child (and probably always will be) who's difficult to get to sleep or placate. But, she is extremely loving, full of fun, very bright and a joy to be with (most of the time!). I love her dearly.

BETTY: AN UNEXPECTED SECOND FAMILY AT 45

Betty, like Helena, became pregnant unintentionally. However, other aspects of her situation were very different. She had been married to Clive for 25 years and they had two children of 19 and 21, a boy and a girl. Betty became pregnant because she had miscalculated her 'safe period', and although she had been to her GP when she realized her mistake it was only with reluctance that he gave her the 'morning after' pill as he said it was extremely unlikely that she would have conceived in view of her advanced age. When Betty found that her fears were confirmed and she was pregnant, despite the pill, she said she was *'really devastated and upset'*. Her husband was shocked because he too had felt that it would be difficult to conceive at their age. Nevertheless he was *'supportive of whatever I chose'*.

Betty had an amniocentesis (*see Chapters 5 and 6*). She said that in view of her circumstances, the Down's blood test *'was not an option really'*, as it would have provided information about the *chances* that her baby had Down's syndrome, but not told her whether or not he or she was *actually* affected. She saw antenatal screening for possible defects as *'a necessary evil'* because it forced her to consider the possibility of terminating the pregnancy, but once she had received the result of her amniocentesis she said: *'I realised I was happy* [to be pregnant] *after the amnio results. I had tried to be detached till then.'*

Betty was well-supported, especially by her husband and daughter, but she did find that pregnancy made her think of her mother who was dead.

> *When my older children were born my mother was still alive. I relied quite heavily upon her for help, advice and support. I have missed her more, recently, since becoming pregnant again than I have for several years and feel saddened by the fact that she will not be around when the baby is born.*

She had been *'a bit worried'* about giving birth but in fact things went very well and she gave the experience *'ten out of ten'*.   Her grown-up children were afraid that they might be woken up at night while the baby was very young, but this turned out not to be a problem because they were themselves fairly nocturnal in their habits! As an aside, Betty also mentioned that things had worked out better than expected even where the family pets were concerned.

> *One cat used to be very demanding. Now that's stopped and he's taken charge – he guards Alex. The other keeps out of the way – she goes out when Alex comes in.*

༂

Planned pregnancies: causes of delay

Unintentional delay: early and late miscarriage

Some 'planned' babies arrive after their mothers are 35, not because the latter have delayed motherhood intentionally, or because they have had problems conceiving, but because they have had one or more miscarriages. The feelings of bereavement and anxiety arising from these experiences can colour the whole experience of subsequent pregnancies, as Janine's story shows.

JANINE: 37, WORRIES ABOUT MISCARRIAGE

People look at me, see some swelling, but are nervous of asking me if I'm pregnant.

Janine's previous miscarriages made everyone concerned for her. Janine was 37 and was on her fourth pregnancy. Her two previous pregnancies had ended in miscarriages but her first had ended happily, in the birth of a little girl, now five years old. After the birth of Emily, Janine and her husband delayed plans for a second child: '*We wanted to enjoy Emily, and it took us a while to adapt to parenthood!*'

Janine had been married for 13 years to her husband, who was eight years older than her and had been married previously. There was a son from the previous marriage who lived with his mother. Janine and her husband had wanted their second baby to be born '*about four years after Emily*' but things hadn't worked out. In the previous year when Janine was 36, she had become pregnant as planned. Anxious about the possibility of something being wrong with the baby, because of her age, she had chosen to have the CVS test (chorionic villus sampling – a technique which enables a small portion of the tissue developing around the placenta to be removed and tested to reveal any abnormalities in the foetus's chromosomes).

9

Janine explained that the CVS actually caused her to miscarry.

The consultant who did it at 10 weeks said it caused the problem. It was to do with him doing it transcervically and attempting to take a sample from the placenta five times.

After the loss of this baby, Janine was anxious to try and conceive again and did so very quickly. Sadly this pregnancy also ended in a miscarriage at 10 weeks due to *'a blighted ovum'*.

The sadness and disappointment of these two miscarriages led them to stop trying for a baby for a few months. But the following year they decided once again to try to add to their family. She felt *'a desperation to be pregnant again'*. Three months later, although *'it seemed like an eternity'*, Janine was pregnant. This time she felt:

very excited, but far more cautious than in my first pregnancy . . . My feelings about this pregnancy have been markedly affected by these miscarriages.

Janine found it hard to believe in her pregnancy to start with – she carried out a home pregnancy test but

I didn't believe this until it was confirmed by the consultant. I was being monitored very closely so I knew logically [about the pregnancy] before I knew emotionally.

This time Janine decided that she would not undergo any invasive tests, such as CVS or amniocentesis, to find out about any chromosomal abnormalities, but despite this she felt, at 37, under some pressure to have these tests even though her history of problems was well known:

there have been frequent suggestions or questions about having these by midwives and other doctors. I feel as though I have to justify myself and say why I'm not. I feel perfectly justified.

The pregnancy was an anxious time for Janine. She repeatedly summed up her feelings as 'cautious' and 'careful'. Despite this worry, all went well and Janine and her husband had a beautiful baby girl. She, they decided, would complete their family.

Summing up her views on antenatal testing and the pros and cons Janine said:

> *I don't like the categorization of females at 35 years and the doubts that that can cause. Having to make those decisions about the results. It's the only time I've envied women in the third world.*

ISABEL: 35, LOSS OF A BABY WITH A CHROMOSOMAL
ABNORMALITY

Isabel's first successful pregnancy was at 35 not by choice but because her earlier pregnancy had ended in a late miscarriage. When asked how much she'd wanted to have this baby she replied:

> *I was absolutely desperate. I was devastated to lose our baby last year and couldn't go back to work when I didn't conceive. I was so upset.*

The second pregnancy had been delayed due to the bereavement they felt following her miscarriage. Before trying to conceive again she and her husband had waited *'until I was physically and emotionally back to normal'*.

Her first baby had died in utero at 20 weeks; one year before our interview. It had been a little girl with Turner's syndrome – a condition in which there is only one sex chromosome instead of the usual two Xs. This condition is characterized by a number of physical features and such females will not menstruate or be able to have a baby. It was not known why the baby died: Turner's syndrome is a genetic condition that does not generally cause death.

Isabel and her husband, who was several years younger, had been married only a couple of years and they had decided before they had married that they wanted children straightaway. Waiting until her thirties to have children seemed natural and obvious to Isabel. She had always wanted children, but *'I wouldn't consider becoming a single parent – intentionally'.*

She wouldn't have had a child outside marriage and had had an abortion in her twenties. The earlier miscarriage had cast something of a shadow over the current pregnancy: *'I've been more tired, anxious and irritable . . . because of last year'.*

Having scans and an amniocentesis had caused a lot of worry. Isabel explained that having a scan made her *'fear that there would be something immediately apparent that was wrong'* and waiting for weeks for the results was particularly nerve-wracking because of *'the fear of the unknown and not knowing what one would do if there was an adverse result'.*

Some months after our interview Isabel had a perfect, healthy, baby boy. They were both fine and all the family very happy. A year later at our last interview Isabel was pregnant again. All went well and she had a perfect baby daughter a few months later.

Intentionally delayed pregnancy

The next two women we describe could be said to have made a conscious decision to wait till their mid-thirties before considering having a child.

ILONA: 35, NOW OR NEVER?

Ilona has just turned 35. She has always assumed that she would have children but until the last year or so had not really wanted to have a baby. Career has always been an important part of her identity. She is an academic and it has taken many years doing higher degrees and working her way up the university career ladder to establish herself at a level at which she feels she can take some time out to have children. Three years ago, at 32, she was promoted to a senior lectureship and felt that she had attained the level of seniority she sought before taking time out – she felt she had established her career. At this time, however, other considerations meant that the time was not right to have a child. Ilona had married at 27. Her husband, Simon, who was three years younger than her, was not then established in a career. He was still training and a full-time student, so Ilona's salary was their sole income. Both Simon and Ilona wanted to buy a house and establish themselves financially before taking on the responsibility and change of lifestyle which comes with having children.

Though Ilona has not had a burning desire to have a child, the pressure of age has made the issue of children more urgent. It is not so much that she considers it 'risky' to have a child later but rather the concern about whether or not she is fertile. There is no history of infertility in her family, but in her late twenties Ilona experienced some hormonal problems for which she had treatment, and this has raised concern that she might have difficulty conceiving. *'I want to know about my fertility so that there is time to sort out any problems before it is too late.'*

Her personal circumstances have also changed. Her husband is now firmly established in his career and she is no longer the primary income earner. The pressures of finances and career are no longer a deterrent.

There are also social pressures.

[Her parents] *talk about their friends becoming grandparents and about children . . . I'm not sure if they always did this and I'm more sensitive to it or whether they've just started to do it.*

Ilona's friends, who had also delayed having children, have now started to have children. Her closest friend had her first child recently, at the age of 34. This has been an important event. It has somehow made pregnancy seem more acceptable and has given her the opportunity to learn more about what pregnancy is like. Until now other people having children has not been significant. What has been important this time is that it is someone close, with the same attitudes and values in life.

When we last spoke to Ilona she had decided, after a long period of debating the pros and cons of children, to go ahead and try to become pregnant.

ANGELA: 35, PLANNED TO PERFECTION

Angela's pregnancy was definitely planned, and like Maureen she experienced very low levels of depression or anxiety, even though her relationship broke up during the pregnancy. She had had an early marriage which broke up 15 years previously and was in a relationship in which she had strong feelings about wanting to get pregnant.

> *We talked a lot about babies. All sorts of feelings welled up very strongly. My age did enter into it because I didn't suppress feelings about* [wanting] *children whereas I had done in the past.*

They planned the pregnancy two weeks before conception. She expected to, and did, conceive at the first 'attempt'.

> *I knew when I was ovulating and we timed conception accordingly . . . We would have kept trying until we both accepted that the relationship wasn't good enough.*

How did other people react?

> *Some of my relatives in their sixties said that termination was the only option for someone in my situation. I was angry . . . what cheek . . . and upset at their selfishness. A few other relatives have made foolish comments . . . but in general people have been really nice; I've been pleasantly surprised. There's a warmth and friendliness I've never felt before.*

She, herself, felt very positive despite the breakdown of her relationship with the baby's father.

> *I feel more able to cope now* [while pregnant] *than ever before. Colleagues at work have helped with things like the physical effort involved in moving house, but I feel more confident now than I was before I was pregnant. With close friends . . . I've become more open; they've become more supportive, and our friendships are stronger.*

Angela returned to work after the birth of her baby, and enjoyed the challenge of combining the roles of mother and worker. Five months after the birth:

Overall life seems much easier since I had Edward. I'm better orga-nized. I do things faster. I make better use of my time: altogether I'm coping better.

And by the time Edward was one:

I work in a male-dominated area. Everything changed in the staff-room when I got pregnant. Now I'm not a threat and they can be friendly, because I'm not 'a single woman' but 'a mother' . . . I know I'm capable of supporting and caring for someone else as well as myself . . . It's also helped sort out how I feel about men and sex. Before Edward was born I went out with men and ended up in bed because that was what you did. No wonder they [relationships] were disas-trous.

She continues to have no contact with Edward's father.

Last time I spoke to him was when I rang him to ask if he wanted me to name him on the birth certificate. He couldn't decide. He's never contacted me since then.

 ✺

One, two, three, four, five . . . or more?

The majority of women who give birth after 35 have already had children, whether many years previously or relatively recently. What issues are important to them in contemplating a 'later' pregnancy? Mary, Shirley and Clare all have different stories to tell.

The 'only child' issue . . .

MARY: 38, SHOULD I HAVE ANOTHER CHILD?

Mary had her first child 18 months ago at the age of 36. She is undecided about having a second child but it is currently an issue about which she thinks a lot and which she intermittently discusses with her husband.

Prior to her first pregnancy Mary had worked for a large company in an administrative job. She had worked there for 15 years and had a good group of friends at work. In their spare time she and her husband, David, renovated the houses they lived in. Their current house was the third they had worked on and their dream home. They did not intend to do up any more houses. Mary had left her job when she started maternity leave.

Her first pregnancy was not a good one. It was marked by serious ill-health requiring a great deal of medical intervention throughout, including hospital stays. These problems culminated in the pre-term delivery of her son at 34 weeks gestation. She and her son recovered well, however, and though she is likely to experience the same problems again they do not really put her off having another. She is undecided because she is content with the one child she has.

Mary and her husband had both wanted a son and were thrilled when James was born. They had both adapted to parenthood well and enjoyed their time with James. They did not have a burning desire to have another child. If they had had a girl first of all they both felt that they would have wanted to 'try for a boy', but they had got what they wanted first time. Having an only child was the issue that concerned them, particularly David, and made them consider trying for a second child. Neither Mary nor David were only children. Mary had a sister and David was one of three boys. Though they did not feel strongly that this had been an important part of their own development they were concerned that James might 'miss out' if he did not have a brother or sister. Mary took James to many local groups where he met other children and so was not isolated in that way, but the concern was that James might be denied something important because everybody else had a brother or sister. There was also pressure from family and friends. From Mary's point of view she was actually content with one but just '*niggled*' by the issue of an only child. Her husband was tending towards wanting a second child. Mary's age and concern about her health put pressure on them to make a decision soon. They feel she has limited time in which to have another. But for now they remain undecided . . .

. . . and larger families

SHIRLEY: SURPRISED BUT HAPPY AT 49

Shirley was 49 when the last of her four children was born. The baby, Peter, arrived 12 years after her previous son, and her whole family arrived over a period of 17 years. Peter's arrival was quite a surprise. Shirley said that when people learned of her late pregnancy it was '*greeted in about equal quantities of incredulity, amusement, pity and envy*'. The baby was not planned but both she and her husband were happy on discovering her pregnancy:

> *We never took 'precautions' as we wanted children but had great difficulty in doing so. We were married seven years before I became pregnant as the result of having progesterone injections. After No. 1 nothing happened again for two and a half years till I took progesterone pills that time and No. 2 immediately started. No. 3 appeared two and a half years later without injections or pills. We took rather haphazard precautions after that as we felt three was enough. When I was 48 I had what the hospital called an abortive pregnancy and a year later Peter arrived, when I was 49. My main worry was that Peter would not be normal . . . I also felt an ass buying maternity clothes!*

The pregnancy was quite straightforward and when compared to her earlier pregnancies Shirley said it was '*much the same – I found the end weeks more exhausting.*'

Her son was perfect and her fears about abnormality unfounded.
   Shirley said that having a son at 49 made her feel younger and

she felt that her son, who was 19 by the time she contacted us, did not mind her being so much older than most mothers. In fact she was surprised that over the whole time she had only twice been mistaken for his grandmother. *'Peter shows no signs of minding, he is a very good companion.'*

Shirley believes that older mothers have special qualities to offer to their children. *'One is lazier and less bound by theories.'* For her the ideal age to become a mother is 35 but she recommends motherhood after 40 too.

I feel having Peter was one of the best things we ever did.

CLARE: 41, FOUR AFTER 35

At 41, Clare was the mother of six children all under the age of ten and four of whom were born to her after her thirty-fifth birthday. Hers was a very straightforward story, the only slight problem was that it took some time for her to conceive her first child.

Although she had always assumed that one day she would have her own family it hadn't been a *'burning factor'* in her life. Clare had trained for some years and was interested in her career as a radiographer and it was not until she'd been in a stable relationship for some time that she began to feel broody, between the ages of 27 and 28. She and her husband started 'trying' but nothing happened. Clare recalled her disappointment each month: *'You'd almost burst into tears every period.'* Despite this it was not until they'd been trying for a baby for three years that Clare sought medical advice on their lack of success. She explained:

> *I'd heard that there was a seven to eight month waiting list before seeing someone, so I went to my GP to get the process started.*

The appointment came sooner than expected, only three to four months after her visit to the GP, and the result of the visit was quite a surprise:

I left the appointment being told I was 15 weeks pregnant. My periods were being irregular. I had spotting every month. I thought, I'm not pregnant – I kept on bleeding. I was vomiting . . . there were lots of bugs going around. I thought it was that and put it down to being tired.

So from there we didn't have any problems.

Clare and her husband, John, were both drawn to the idea of a large family as neither had come from one themselves. Asked about how many children she wanted:

Initially I thought four. The idea of six at the outset had not occurred but after each baby then we felt another one would be nice.

Although commenting '*I'm never well with a pregnancy*' Clare didn't see age as having any influence on the first four pregnancies and births which she described as normal. In her last two pregnancies she noted '*I had to be a bit more careful and rest more*', but she was not at all certain that this was due to her age, pointing out that the presence of four or five young children around the home to care for might have been the crucial difference between her earlier and later pregnancies.

When asked whether age was an issue to those around her she replied:

No, nobody had ever suggested that . . . or made a comment that I was too old to have babies. [The consultant laughed at her last pregnancy and] *he said I was a grandmultip because I was on my sixth pregnancy.*

Are more babies planned?

I've said no . . . because of my age. I'd be 42 if I had it straight away. I'd be 62 by the time it was 20 . . . I don't want to be drawing my pension and my child benefit at the same time. We've been lucky, you see. All the children are healthy. I feel . . . we should stop while we're ahead.

And her husband?

. . . at the moment he's after another dog.

୬

These case studies have illustrated the variety of women who become mothers after 35. The accounts raise many issues: planned and unplanned pregnancy, fertility after 35, issues surrounding tests for abnormality during pregnancy, decisions about family size, one or two parent families, combining paid work with motherhood, and the pros and cons of a 'generation gap' of 35-plus years; to mention but a few. The remainder of the book delves more deeply into research on these and other topics.

✤ 2 ✤

Who Has Babies after 35?
Facts and Figures

Having babies after 35 is on the increase. The number of babies born to women aged between 35 and 39 over the last decade has risen more than for any other age group. Indeed in most younger age groups the number of babies born has *decreased*. Yet there are now nearly 50 per cent more babies being born to women aged 35–39 years than at the start of the 1980s in England and Wales.[1,2] This trend is also apparent in the United States and Australia.[3,4,5]

Why are women having their babies later? What factors account for this trend and what sorts of women start, or add to, their families at this stage in life?

In the middle of the twentieth century first-time mothers were younger than today but the pattern of first births in a woman's early twenties was not typical of earlier times. According to Peter Laslett, children in the West always seem to have been born of 'mature women'; by this he means women in their late twenties or their early thirties. Thus the average age for childbirth – currently 27.9 years – is nothing new.[6,1] Giving birth at a later age appears to be more typical of Western family patterns over the last few hundred years than at the early ages for births reported in the 1950s and 1960s.

Influences on the timing of motherhood have changed dramatically during the twentieth century. In this chapter we shall explore how changes in attitudes towards women's education and employment, birth control, marriages, partnerships and single mothers all play an important role in shaping who has babies, but of course the most fundamental issue is a woman's capacity to reproduce: her fecundity. This may be a key factor in influencing the likelihood of a later baby.

∽

The capacity to have babies

Do all women have the potential to bear children at the age of 35 or over? The capacity to reproduce – to be fruitful – is hard to assess, yet we know that today a woman's chances of having a baby later are probably better than at any other time in history. Record ages for births are surprisingly high as can be seen in Box 2.1.

Most young women take it for granted that they are fecund – that they will become pregnant if they try to do so. Establishing that this is so without putting it to the test is less easy – yet there are some basic facts about the capacity to reproduce that we can report.

From first to last menstruation

The menarche, the onset of periods, is taken by most as the beginning of a woman's reproductive life, and the menopause – the last menstruation – is taken to be the end, but around both these events the likelihood of becoming pregnant is much lower than we might expect. It has been suggested that many young girls are anovulatory (not shedding eggs) during the first year or two after menarche and similarly the cycles in the latter stages of reproductive life may also not be fertile.[7,8] Thus from the girl's or woman's point of view her knowledge of her body and her menstrual cycle will not tell her if she will, in fact, conceive.

Comparing women today with women in the past we see that the period over which women are capable of having children has also changed. Since the last century there has been a 'spectacular decline' in the age of first menstruation in the Western world

---

OLDER MOTHERS: A FEW STATISTICS (BOX 2.1)

The oldest mother ever recorded in Britain was Mrs Ellen Ellis of Wales, who gave birth to a stillborn baby, her thirteenth child, in 1776 when she was 72 years of age; this is unauthenticated.[37]

The oldest recorded mother in America was Mrs Ruth Alice Kistler of Portland, Oregon. She gave birth to a daughter on 18 October 1956 when her age was 57 years, 129 days. This record had satisfactory medical verification.[37]

Mrs Kathleen Campbell of Nottingham broke the record for authenticated births in the UK in 1987 by having her eighth child when she was aged 55 years, 141 days. Campbell's record has since been broken by a great grandmother who gave birth at age 59 to her thirteenth child in 1990 according to the *British Medical Journal*.[36]

The oldest mother to give birth by egg donation is Mrs Rosanna Della Corte who gave birth to a baby boy on 18 July 1994 when she was aged 62 years.[40]

In England and Wales in the 1960s the average age for married women to have a first baby was 24 years. Currently the average age for all births is 27.9 years and for married women, 29.1 years.[2]

In England and Wales in the early 1990s, 50 or more babies were born to mothers aged 50 and over each year. In addition, there are about 20 legal abortions per year to women in this age group.[2]

In the late 1930s women were more likely to have babies later in life than they are today. Four per cent of births were to mothers aged 40 and over; 15 per cent were to mothers aged 35 and older.[24]

Most recent Birth Statistics for England and Wales show 9.7 per cent of births are to mothers aged 35 and over and 1.5 per cent are to mothers aged 40 and over.[2]

Over 99 per cent of babies born to mothers aged 40 do not have Down's syndrome (*see chapter 5*).

---

with an average age of menarche of around 12.4 to 13.5 years.[9] In the 1800s in the developed world, girls reached puberty around the age of 16 to 18 and this decline in age is probably due chiefly to the fact that children have been getting progressively taller and heavier at any given age – due mainly to improved nutrition and health.[10]

At the other end of a woman's reproductive life it appears that the age of menopause has changed over the last century, by an estimated increase of four years, but it is hard to establish how true this is.[11] Today the menopause occurs at around 50 in England or 51 in America.[12] At the turn of the century women's life expectancy was less than 50 and thus mortality rates distort the calculations because the deaths of women who would have reached the menopause at a later age are *excluded* from such estimates, unlike those whose menopause was earlier. Nevertheless the timing of motherhood has been extended at the bottom and possibly at the top of the age span so that the modern woman has the potential to bear children over a longer period.

Moreover, as the average family size decreases a woman's likelihood of having had many children by 35 is less than formerly. A woman at 35 contemplating pregnancy today is physically in better shape than her forebears were likely to have been, simply because there has been less physical toll on her body of many previous pregnancies. As George Maroulis has said of those in more developed societies:

> women in their early 40s are young, and although the risk of infertility increases with age it may be modified by fertility drugs, good nutrition, avoidance of infection and so forth.[13]

ॐ

Fertility statistics:
the numbers of babies born

Whilst the potential to have children spans decades, fertility rates – the actual number of babies born – show that the timing of motherhood is shaped by the culture into which a woman is born.

National birth statistics reveal a wide variety of different trends – in the onset, timing, and the cessation of births as well as the number of children born. These sorts of patterns vary greatly over historical time and as was indicated at the start of this chapter many factors play a significant role in determining when women have their children. George Maroulis identifies three key areas of influence: Firstly, intrinsic ageing: by this he means the changes that occur as a result of the biological processes observed as we get older; secondly, weathering, the factors that affect our reproductive system such as infections, smoking and obesity; and thirdly, our history.[13] This latter category is our major concern here since Chapter 5 will deal with becoming pregnant at 35-plus, but history, which includes environmental, social and financial conditions at different historical times, influences recorded 'age-specific fertility rates'. We shall consider some of these factors in explaining recorded birth statistics more fully.

The most fertile people: the Hutterites

There are very few populations in which there is no attempt made to control births – this is particularly so today when contraception is widely available. In the past it was more common for relatively few limits to be placed on reproduction in marriage, but the age of marriage could be one effective way of limiting childbearing at a time when childbirth outside marriage was a considerable stigma.

Fertility statistics from natural populations, with relatively few or no restrictions on fertility, come from historical data and from a few selected groups of contemporary women: one well-researched group is the North American Hutterites, and these people will be considered in detail.[14]

It has been said of the Hutterite population that it: 'is reproducing itself close to the theoretical maximum level of human fertility for all but the 15 – 19 year age group.' The Hutterites are an anabaptist religious sect, living in the United States and Canada. They are a particularly interesting natural population on which to draw since there are complete censuses of the entire population for June 1880 and 31 December 1950. Throughout the entire population there is a high degree of homogeneity in socio-economic status, educational level and other social attributes. Between 1880 and 1950 the sect increased in size *over 19 times* in this 70 year period.

One way of showing the high fertility of this group is to consider the *Fertility Ratio* – this is the number of children under five years of age per 100 women aged between 15 and 49 years (*see Table 2.1*).

Table 2.1. Fertility ratio of the Hutterites and selected populations

Population	Children under 5 years of age per 100 females aged 15–49 years
Hutterites (1948)	96.3
Algeria (Moslems) (1948)	63.1
Jamaica (1949)	49.5
Israel (1948)	45.8
United States (1950)	42.3

Source: Eaton and Mayer, 1953[14]

The figure of 96.3 children under five years old per 100 women in the Hutterites *is greater* than for any other population. It tells us that virtually all women aged between 15 and 49 in this population have at least one small child in their care and this figure can be viewed as an underestimate because very few women marry (or have children) under the age of 19 years.

Virtually all the population marries – by the age of 45 only one per cent of either sex has never been married – and regularity in exposure to pregnancy appears to be accepted as normal in marriage. Thus this is one of the best examples of natural human fertility. There are no general customs that inhibit sex relations in those who are married except for a few weeks before the birth of a baby and for about six weeks afterwards. Outside marriage sexual relations are severely frowned upon and babies born out of wedlock are very rare.

Peak fertility for married Hutterite women seems to be in their twentieth year when 61.1 per cent had a live birth; after this fertility declines progressively but the decline is not pronounced until about the age of 40. It then approaches zero at age 49. Nevertheless statistics for the number of children still possible after a given age show that a few are born to women over 50 (*see Table 2.2*).

Table 2.2 Number of children still possible per woman after any given age by five year age groups for the ethnic Hutterite women alive on 31 December 1950

Age	Number of live births still possible
50	0.02
45	0.19
40	1.24
35	3.21
30	5.46
25	8.00
20	10.82

(As most women married in their twenties estimates for women under 20 are not given.)

Source: Eaton & Mayer, 1953[14]

The Hutterite population can be viewed as 'a modern population in their death rates . . . but "primitive" in their birth rates'. As a group they live under technological conditions that give a growing population good economic and medical support. The Hutterites place much value on having children and parents receive considerable economic and social support to give adequate care to their children.

Despite very high fertility rates for older women, with a sizeable number born even to those in their fifties, George Maroulis warns that even these figures may *underestimate* the true capacity of women to bear children in these upper age groups, since older women with large families may be less eager to get pregnant, the frequency of intercourse may have diminished in older couples, and problems such as pelvic infections, more frequent in older women, may influence 'inherent biological ability' to get pregnant.[13]

The Hutterite women show us the best example of women's capacity to bear children across their reproductive lives. But in the West the women who have babies after the age of 35 today are not typical of average age mothers. Statistics from past times reveal some significant changes in childbearing patterns.

Fertility statistics in the past

In past times when methods of contraception were much more limited and less reliable, births to older mothers were much more common in Britain and America than they are today. In the 1920s it is said that the average age at which a woman in the US had her last child was 42 years and certainly the continuation of child-bearing into the latter part of the reproductive years was common elsewhere. In Scotland 19 per cent of births in 1855 were to women aged 35 and over.[15] No equivalent statistics are available from England and Wales since age-specific fertility rates were not kept until the 1930s – but first records at that time show that 15 per cent of births were to mothers aged 35 and over. Statistics for Ireland in the 1950s and 1960s show that about one quarter of births were to women aged 35 and over – yet this figure has declined in recent years. In the 1980s only about 16 per cent of births were to this age group.[16,17]

Comparisons between fertility statistics in different age groups tell us little about the likelihood of a woman's capacity to bear children at that age. The frequency of unprotected intercourse is a significant factor here because, in general, those who have had a longer partnership or marriage tend to show a lower rate of inter-course and hence the likelihood of conception is reduced because the fertile period in each cycle is more likely to be missed. Current statistics show that only a small proportion of older women are having babies but this pattern has not remained stable over the last decade or so.

Current fertility statistics

In England and Wales new motherhood for women aged 35 and over is on the increase and this age group is the fastest growing group of new mothers.[1,2] Table 2.3 shows the proportion of live births by age group in England and Wales and indicates that the majority of births are still to women in their twenties with approximately as many teenage births as births to women aged 35 and over. The average age for all births is currently 27.9 years, for all births (in marriage) it is 29.1 years and for first births in marriage it is 27.8 years.[2] This latter figure is the highest *ever* in England and Wales since records began in the 1930s.[18] In the 1960s the average age for first births was 24 years.[19] In Australia the median age for first births (in marriage) was 23 years in the late 1960s and this had increased to 27.6 years by 1990.[5]

Table 2.3. Percentage of live births in England and Wales, by maternal age, born to women in 1992

Age of Mother	Under 20	20–29	30–34	35–39	40 and over
Percentage* of live births	6.9	60.2	24.2	8.2	1.5

*Figures rounded to one decimal point
Adapted from *Birth Statistics*, 1992. HMSO (1994)[2]

A similar trend towards later motherhood has also been recorded in the United States. US births to women aged 30 and over have doubled since 1970.[4] US birth rates show that whilst general fertility has changed very little since the mid-1970s the increase reported for women in their thirties and early forties reflects 'the continuing trend of women postponing childbearing to increasingly older ages'.[3]

Research shows that women who become mothers later, particularly first-time mothers, have particular characteristics in terms of their education, occupation, partnerships, marriages or lack of these, and fertility history, and we shall now consider in detail these features of present-day older mothers.

꒰ᔅ꒱

Education and occupation

One factor that appears to influence the timing of motherhood is a woman's education and her choice of paid work. Jane Wilkie has observed that delaying motherhood . . . 'is a recent strategy adopted by women interested in careers, especially those with higher education.'[20] The role of education has been highlighted strongly by Ronald Rindfuss who has suggested that each additional year of schooling has resulted in a delay of about nine months for the first birth.[21] This tendency to delay looks as if it can only increase in view of the increased number of women in higher education and in the workforce. There is no doubt that childbearing and childrearing can have an adverse effect on women's employment and it has been pointed out that these events cost a woman up to one-half of her potential life-time's earnings.[22]

A number of researchers have found that older first-time mothers are more likely to be in the professions and to be highly educated. Iris Kern reported this for an American sample of older mothers and a similar situation was found in studies by two of the authors, Julia Berryman and Kate Windridge.[23] In this sample of 346 British 40-plus mothers, 80 per cent of first-time mothers were from non-manual or professional occupations, whereas rather less (about half) of those with previous children were categorized in this way.[24] In the Leicester Motherhood Project also carried out by two of the authors all the first-time 35-plus mothers recruited were also in non-manual occupations and many were in the professions.[25] Despite this, a conscious delaying of a pregnancy for career reasons was not necessarily part of the explanation given for opting for a later baby. In the 40-plus sample of mothers only 5 per cent gave 'career reasons' as an explanation for their later baby.

As women are expected to participate more fully in the work-force throughout their lives, and as more enter higher education, it is no surprise that the timing of motherhood is likely to be influenced. Schools, colleges and universities are not settings which combine well with motherhood – at least in their present form – and similarly, in a patriarchal world, most of the professions are designed with males rather than females in mind. Choosing when to fit in motherhood is problematic when promotion is put in jeopardy. If, and when, such occupations are changed to allow a more flexible approach to career breaks, women will then have more choice about when to start a family.

ॐ

Birth control

Women have always had some degree of control over whether or not to have children. In the past marriage was a significant means of control and the delay of marriage was one means of reducing the number of pregnancies in a woman's lifetime. Once married the rate of intercourse and methods such as coitus interruptus may have helped space pregnancies where no other means were available.

At such times the incidence of later babies was more a reflection of a women's fecundity than are fertility statistics today. In 1950, the probability of having another baby for a 45-year-old Hutterite woman was nearly one in 10; currently in England and Wales the likelihood of a baby being born to a woman of 35 and over is the same – nearly one in 10.

Effective reproductive control through contraception has been available now for some decades and with the arrival of oral contraceptives – 30 or so years ago – women have had much greater freedom of choice over the timing of their families. In Great Britain whilst the pill is the most popular method of contraception in the under 35s, for women aged 35 and over sterilization is the most commonly chosen method (22 per cent).[18] Amongst men in this age group there is a very similar situation:

23 per cent of over 35s are sterilized. Whilst we cannot assume that these men are in partnership with women of the same age it is likely that amongst older women a good proportion of births are prevented by either female or male sterilization.

After sterilization, use of the male condom is the next method of choice in the over 35s. This age group is also most likely to be using contraception (76 per cent use some method), compared with an overall figure for contraceptive use at 70 per cent. In spite of this the use of contraception is still somewhat patchy and, if abortion statistics are anything to go by, there are many babies that are conceived, by women of all ages, who are not destined to be born. Whilst abortion statistics don't tell us that a baby was unplanned – some planned pregnancies may be terminated because of foetal abnormalities or because partnerships break down after the conception – they give some guide to pregnancies that have arisen through failure or lack of adequate contraception.

Anne Fleissig, in a recent paper on 'unintended' pregnancies, reports that approximately one third of babies born fall into this category.[26] This does not mean that they are unwanted children but it reflects something about today's contraceptive practices. Of course many unintended pregnancies become abortions and the abortion figures show that relative to the age of the mother the proportion of terminations to births are greatest in the very young and the 'very old' expectant mother.

Until 1982 in England and Wales more pregnancies were terminated in women aged 40 and over than were followed through to full-term.[1] The only other age group where this high termination rate was found was in girls aged under 16. Thus in the much older mother unintended pregnancies appear to be particularly high. Perhaps this reflects the expectations of women in their forties that a pregnancy is very unlikely. Certainly in the British study of 40-plus mothers *less than half* the babies were planned and a few pregnancies were mistaken for the menopause.

This apparent lack of planning in the woman in her forties does not seem to be reflected in the mother in her early thirties. A number of studies suggest that the majority of mothers at this stage are planning their families.[1,27,28] Most or all women in their thirties in two quite different studies were found to have voluntarily postponed childbearing unlike those in their twenties where less conscious choices seemed to have been made.

In an American sample of mothers in their late thirties studied by Iris Kern, only half of the babies were planned, whereas in the Leicester Motherhood Project two thirds of the sample of mothers aged 35 and over were 'trying' to get pregnant.[23] Younger women in their twenties showed a similar trend except that even more first-time mothers were 'trying' to get pregnant (88 per cent).

ॐ

Marriages and partnerships

Are later babies more common nowadays because there are more second marriages? It certainly is the case that there are more divorces and remarriages today in the West than in earlier times. Over a third of marriages in Britain are remarriages for at least one partner, and all but two per cent of these are remarriages due to a previous divorce. In Britain this figure has risen dramatically; thirty years ago less than one in 10 marriages was a remarriage.[18] In America the proportion of remarriages to marriages is even higher.[29]

Married before?

In the Leicester Motherhood Project it was the case that more of the older (over 35) than the younger (20 – 29) group had been married before.[25] Nearly 30 per cent of the over 35s had been married before whereas only one in 20 of the younger women had, and a previous marriage was more likely in both age groups amongst the mothers who had one or more previous children. In both samples the first-time mothers had been in their current marriage or partnership for a shorter time than had those women, in either age group, who had previous children. In the

American study Iris Kern found a similar pattern; 28 per cent of her sample of mothers aged between 35 and 43 were in a second marriage when their 'later' baby was born.[23]

Younger partners

One rather unexpected finding that emerged from examining the partnerships of older mothers in both British studies by the authors was the increased likelihood of such a mother having a younger partner.

Amongst women in the British study of 40-plus mothers it was found that mothers of first-borns had partners who were on average *three years younger* than they were: a notable finding in view of the fact that husbands are generally an average of two and a half years older than their wives.[24] The Leicester Motherhood Project revealed a similar but less pronounced trend in the sample of women aged 35 and over.[25] First-time mothers aged 35 and over differed significantly from the other three groups in our study (older mothers of more than one child, or younger mothers between 20–29 years having their first-born, or having more than one child). Unlike the other groups older first-time mothers' partners were nearly a year younger on average than they were, whereas all the other age groups had partners older on average than the women themselves.

Thus the first-time mother who is older than average is likely to be in a relationship of shorter duration, is more likely to have had a previous marriage and is more likely to have a younger partner.

ॐ

Lone mothers

The lone mother is not usually pictured as a woman in her thirties or forties but for those 'up against the clock' there may be a keen need to have a child, with or without a partner, before it is too late. Single mothers are often thought of as those who 'made a mistake' – younger women, perhaps teenage girls, who are ignorant of contraception or have simply allowed themselves to get pregnant without consciously choosing motherhood. In Britain and America much wrath has been directed against these younger mothers because they gain various state benefits, or state housing ahead of those viewed as in *real* need. Without wishing to debate these issues it is perhaps time to readjust our ideas of the lone mother. Today many women are the sole carers of their children and amongst those who become mothers later an increasing number go ahead without a regular partner.

The feeling that the biological clock is ticking away can start well before the mid-thirties. As Anna, approaching thirty, put it:

> *Time is running out and motherhood is something I believe myself to be particularly well suited to, so I'll just have to get on with it on my own.*[30]

Anna went on to conceive by donor insemination and found, when she went to a private clinic for treatment, that about 10 per cent of the women there were single like her.

A fifth of births to women over 35 are outside marriage in England and Wales and the number has doubled in 10 years. Of course not all these women lack partners but it is likely that many of them do. Our research supports this contention – nearly 10 per cent of the 35-plus sample in the Leicester Motherhood Project were without a partner and some of our 40-plus mothers were too.[24,25] Concern over this trend has been widely expressed in the media in articles such as 'Women who want the baby but not the man' but whatever our personal views the trend is increasing and there is evidence that many people are not unduly concerned: a recent survey revealed that '48 per cent of the population believe that a single mother can bring up her child as well as a married couple'.[31]

~

Do fertility problems precede later babies?

Are later babies just the result of trying for a baby for much longer than average? One obvious explanation for the 35-plus baby is that the advances in reproductive technology in recent decades have been so great that women who had abandoned hope of a child in their mid-twenties could 10, or even 20 years later (between 1970 and 1990), find that a new treatment has appeared that might suit them.

Prior to the arrival of the test-tube baby technique (in-vitro fertilization) women whose Fallopian tubes were blocked had to abandon hope of their own child. But in 1978, the world's first test-tube baby, Louise Brown, was born following the pioneering work of Patrick Steptoe and Robert Edwards, and thus the test-tube technique became an option for a group of women who probably thought that motherhood had eluded them.[32]

After this, other procedures such as GIFT – Gamete Intra-Fallopian Transfer – enabled more and more of those previously thought to be unable to get pregnant to do so. GIFT is a technique that achieves a conception rate higher than that of normal intercourse around ovulation. It is thus well suited to those whose infertility is unexplained or for those whose fertility was known to be declining – as in the woman in her late thirties or early forties. IVF and GIFT are discussed further in Chapter 4.

Egg donation has also become an option for women who do not have their own eggs – such as those suffering from Turner's syndrome (a condition in which a woman lacks one sex chromosome and is infertile) and, as we shall see later, a technique has been developed to enable those who have gone through the menopause (early or at the usual age) to achieve a pregnancy. Between 10 and 15 per cent of couples have a fertility problem and we would expect this figure to increase the longer couples wait before trying to achieve a pregnancy.[33] Thus couples in their early twenties will on average achieve a conception more quickly than those in their thirties or early forties.

If there is a general shift amongst the whole population

towards delaying the starting of families then this will have an effect on the numbers seeking fertility treatment. The numbers of older women having sought fertility advice or treatment are well above the average for the population in general. Forty per cent of the mothers, or two in every five women in our study who had a baby at 40 or over, sought help or advice for fertility problems.[24] There was also a much greater range of time taken to conceive their infant. One mother, for example, had waited 26 years for her much-wanted baby born when she was 47.

ॐ

The 50-plus mother: naturally or not

Even now women giving birth after 50 are the cause of interest and comment (if they admitted to their age), because for the majority biology has called 'time'. The average age for the last menstruation is around 50 and fertility is known to be very low approaching the menopause. As was noted the Hutterite women are amongst the most fertile, but all countries have examples of the 50-plus new mothers. For example, in 1990 in England and Wales there were 58 births and 21 legal abortions in those aged 50 or more.[34] In Britain, Kathleen Campbell, aged 55, gave birth to a son in 1987 and at that time became the British record holder. She was the mother of seven other children, the last of whom was born 16 years previously.[35] Mrs Campbell upset certain presumptions made in English law since 'Section 2 of the Perpetuities and Accumulations Act 1964' states that a female who has attained the age of 55 will not be able to have a child.[36] Since Mrs Campbell a number of other even older mothers have been reported in Britain. Harini Narayan and others studied seven women who have given birth over 50 between 1989 and 1990 in a hospital in Birmingham, England.[37] All the women had many previous children (range five to twelve per woman) and had 63 prior pregnancies between them, of which there were two preterm deliveries and 59 full-term vaginal deliveries, including two sets of twins. The oldest woman of the group had had a previous baby less than one year before the birth that was studied and the latter occurred when she was 59. All the women were first generation Asian Muslims originally from either Pakistan or Bangladesh. One of the world's oldest women ever to give birth is thought to be Mrs Ellen Ellis, of Four Crosses, Clwyd, Wales who allegedly, at the age of 72, had a still-born baby on 15 May 1776.[38] This case is unauthenticated.

In addition to these natural pregnancies there is now the new phenonemon of the older mother who has achieved a pregnancy after the menopause by egg donation. In America, Michal Sauer has assisted a number of women to achieve a pregnancy successfully, and in Italy Severino Antinori is renowned for such treatment in women over 50; he claims that he has helped more than 70 women to give birth after the menopause.[39,40] The women who have sought such treatment are not necessarily childless. The American singer Joni Mitchell gave birth in her fifties to a baby by this procedure; she has four of her own children by her first marriage and a young adopted daughter with her new husband. She also had two grandchildren and a third on the way when she became pregnant by egg donation.[41] Her wish for a sibling for her adopted daughter, Sydney, led her and her husband to seek a baby by egg donation. Other well known cases include an Italian woman, Rosanna Della Corte, who sought treatment following the loss of her only son in a motor-scooter accident at the age of 17, and three years later gave birth to a baby boy on 18 July 1994 at the age of 62; also a 59 year-old British woman who gave birth to twins in 1993. Both women received treatment from Severino Antinori.[39]

Little can be said collectively about the characteristics of these older mothers – their motives seem to be as varied as those of any other group. They have given rise to much worldwide debate about the rights of women to give birth after the natural deadline and the possible need to legislate to reduce or prevent such treatments. Later in this book we shall discuss women's attitudes to postmenopausal treatments of this type.

∽ 3 ∽

Why Have Babies after 35?
Decision-making and
Later Parenthood

Perhaps the greatest contribution to the recent trend towards delayed parenthood outlined in Chapter 2 are the advances in contraceptive and reproductive technology. Contraception has allowed couples to decide not to become parents at all, to plan more precisely when to have children and to limit family size. Reproductive technology on the other hand has presented the possibility of parenthood to those who would previously have remained involuntarily childless. These new technologies present the possibility of control and developing alongside them has been a social expectation that this control will be exercised.[1] Planning of parenthood and restriction of family size has increasingly become viewed as socially responsible. Economic and career pressures and the social expectation that women should be part of the workforce present further issues for consideration before becoming a parent. More than ever before women, and men, are directed to make decisions about parenthood. As having a baby after 35 is part of a whole range of decisions about motherhood, in this chapter we examine the factors affecting decisions about parenthood in general before particularly considering those that lead to motherhood after the age of 35. We examine the decision to become a mother, the factors affecting the timing of first-time motherhood, and finally the decision about subsequent children and their spacing.

ᘓ

Choosing Motherhood

Is motherhood inevitable?

It has been argued that there is an innate biological drive to reproduce and therefore parenthood is not so much a choice but an inevitable life stage. This is difficult to prove but clearly there are psychological and social pressures which direct women, in particular, towards the choice of parenthood.

PSYCHOLOGICAL PRESSURES – MOTHERHOOD AS MANDATORY

Most women assume that they will become a mother at some stage in their reproductive life. Studies of young women indicate that, for the majority, parenthood is part of a general life plan.[2,3,4] A recent study by Heather Wallach and Margaret Maitlin, for example, found that 68 per cent of women (average age 18 years 9 months) described themselves as extremely likely to have children and also had firm views on the number of children they would have, with most expecting to have two.[2]

Studies of women experiencing fertility problems provide more powerful evidence of the unspoken expectation of parenthood.[5,6] The discovery of a fertility problem challenges a life plan that for most is taken for granted until this point. Ann Woollett[5] reports that women who have experienced fertility problems and those who are childless by choice, because they do not conform to common reproductive patterns and because they are often required to articulate their ideas about motherhood, are more conscious of the values surrounding motherhood. Women experiencing fertility problems report a sense of loss and anger at being cheated out of an experience that is rightfully theirs, as the following words from Julia Berryman's study of women awaiting egg donation convey:

I felt cheated. I felt it was my right to choose whether to have a baby. That choice was taken away from me.[7]

Angela, 40, no children

As well as feeling angry or desolate at my plight of being unable to conceive after all these years I also feel angry at the system and the doctors who treat us who don't always make things clear, who waste our time and our reserve tank of hope.

Jane, 40, no children

They also describe a sense of being excluded from adult female identity:

Feeling broody is a deep yearning which I try to control because, since an operation in 1974 leaving me unable to have children, I often feel guilty, sometimes stupid. Feeling broody also makes me feel inadequate amongst other people.

Jenny, 40, no children

I felt like a barren woman before. Now I feel more feminine.

Ruth, 36, on conceiving after trying for 12 years

Clearly, becoming a parent is, for most women, a normal developmental stage and the fulfilment of an important life role.

SOCIAL PRESSURES: JOINING THE CLUB

Becoming a parent is also a social norm. The expectations of other individuals and groups are likely to influence women's choices in favour of having children. Religious affiliation is a factor influencing some but more commonly parents and peers are those most likely to assert social pressure. Women and their partners may experience direct pressure from parents who want to continue the family line and become grandparents. Those who are only children, whose parents or parents-in-law do not already have grandchildren or whose parents are elderly may feel particular pressure – a duty to fulfill family expectation.

Friends are also likely to exert indirect pressure. Maxine Soloway and Rebecca Smith report that in their study of couples who had children later, friends had an influence on preventing parenthood before the age of 30 but after that time they were a positive influence as the values of the group changed.[8] Once members of a social group have children the activities and lifestyle of the group inevitably change. As a consequence there is a pressure to conform – remaining part of the group may mean taking the decision to have children too. Friends with children may also present an acceptable model of parenthood and make the choice more desirable. They convey the message that 'it is all right to become a parent' and provide the opportunity for first hand contact with children that may not be available elsewhere.

In the Australian Timing of Motherhood study by one of the authors, Karen Thorpe, and Jana Cinnamon factors affecting the decision to become a mother were examined among 140 Australian women who had given birth to their first child at a time early (under 25 years), average (between 25 and 29 years) or late (30 years and over) relative to the national birth figures.[9] Individual circumstances and feelings were identified as most prominent in the decision to become a parent – these were the more obvious foreground issues. However, pressure from family, pressure from friends and the example of others having children were portrayed as underlying, background influences. Of these three, the positive example of others having children was the most influential, though for older women family pressure was also an issue. It would seem that while direct pressure from others may be felt, familiarity with parenthood afforded by the experience of other people's children makes parenthood a more acceptable and desirable option.

The immediate network of family and friends is not the only source of social influence: Ann Woollett[5] and Ann Oakley[10] both report that motherhood is seen as a socially acceptable role and failure to become a mother as unacceptable.[4,10] It is also a source of new friendships based on shared experience. For those who have children it is a 'club' from which those unable to have children may feel excluded – 'the freemasonry of the fertile'.[10,11]

In summary, there are possibly biological and certainly

psychological and social pressures that make it more likely that a woman will make a choice to have children. These pressures are best described as personal and social expectations which underlie the decision whether or not to become a parent. In the foreground are personal assessments of the benefits and costs of becoming a parent.

The costs of motherhood

Becoming a mother presents not only the acquisition of a new role but also the loss or change of others. Primary amongst the costs that might influence the decision to become a mother are its negative impact on career, finances, personal freedom and lifestyle.

CAREER RETARDATION

Having a child inevitably alters or interrupts career development. Motherhood brings with it a diversion of roles and responsibility that limits the time and energy that might formerly have been directed solely to career. Whether a choice is made to continue work, and whether this be on a full or part-time basis, having a child is likely to slow career development and limit working hours. Prospects for promotion are likely to be affected because of this.[12,13,14] Many women find that either by choice or organizational decision they are given less demanding roles on return to work.[15,16] The under-representation of women in senior levels of many career structures clearly reflects the impact of childbearing.[16,17]

FINANCIAL COST

Having a child presents a double financial burden. Firstly, there is that associated with changed patterns of paid work and the cost of daycare. Income is lost if a woman decides to cease paid work or reduce the number of paid hours of work. For those hours that the woman does work costs are typically incurred for daycare. These are often considerable and may account for a large proportion of her salary.[16,17] Secondly, the child presents costs in its own right. The long-term financial costs of feeding, clothing and educating a child, though difficult to quantify, are considerable and will certainly have an impact on disposable income and lifestyle. It has been estimated that child-bearing and childrearing can cost up to half a woman's lifetime earnings.[18] The financial cost of children is sometimes given as the reason for delay, as women more developed in their career earn relatively more, more easily cover the additional costs and have more control of earning.

LOSS OF PERSONAL FREEDOM

The care of a child, particularly in the first year of life, is very demanding and may limit women's lifestyle in terms of both range and spontaneity of activities. Previous leisure pursuits may not be feasible with a young child and the physical demands of care may reduce energy levels. Though having a child also creates opportunities to engage in new activities, the loss of lifestyle is often presented as a cost of parenthood. Susan Bram reports in her study which compared couples who were already parents, intending to have children later, or voluntarily childless, that loss of spontaneity and unwanted additional responsibility were important factors which distinguished the groups. Those who intended to remain childless placed greatest emphasis on personal freedom.[19] A study of 80 women in the United States identified the loss of personal freedom as the major theme underlying delaying parenthood.[20] In the Australian Timing of Motherhood study mothers were asked to describe the most difficult aspects of being a mother.[9] The most common theme across all age groups was the loss of personal freedom and lifestyle:

> *What is so difficult is the baby's complete attachment to me . . . the 24 hour responsibility.*
>
> > *Julie, 32, mother of one child aged 10 months*

When I was pregnant I thought I would do lots of projects – sewing,
reading, gardening – as I was only going to be working part-time.
What is so difficult and frustrating is that not only can I not do these
things but I can't even do the everyday things that I used to do. Jobs are
never finished, I never get time to myself – not even to go to the toilet
or have a shower. Unfortunately, children don't have an off button.

Alice, 34, mother of one child aged nine months

IMPACT ON RELATIONSHIP WITH PARTNER

Change in the relationship between the couple is also a likely
consequence of parenthood. Having a child may have an adverse
effect on the sexual relationship in the first year after birth. A
recent survey by the National Childbirth Trust (NCT) found
that sex life was worse for 50 per cent of couples during this
time.[21] Lack of sleep and the impact of breastfeeding in reducing
libido were the major contributants to reduced sexual activity.
Other aspects of relationship may also be affected. Some women
experience poor emotional well-being following childbirth and
this may adversely affect the quality of relationship with partner.[22]
Reduced quality of relationship is not necessarily a consequence
of having a child, however. Indeed for some it is the focus for
improvement. In Susan Bram's study those who were not yet
parents, particularly those who intended to remain childless,
were more likely to perceive the effects of a child on the relationship with partner as negative.[19] Thus for women who delay
becoming a mother concerns about adverse effects on the relationship with their partner may be a more important issue. The
impact of a baby on the relationship with a partner is discussed
further in chapter 7.

The benefits of motherhood

Having a child opens up a whole new world of experience and
change of relationships. The benefits of having children are
perhaps less tangible than the costs. In the Australian Timing of

Motherhood study mothers were asked to describe the rewards of being a mother.[9] The responses given did not differ according to the age of the mother at the birth but rather were common to all women. These could be broadly categorized as: development of relationships, personal fulfilment and achievement, and genetic immortality.

DEVELOPMENT OF RELATIONSHIPS

Becoming a mother is often a turning point in the development of existing relationships and the source of new, positive relationships. When asked about the most rewarding aspects of motherhood one mother in the Australian Timing of Motherhood study replied:

> *just the love and affection I receive from my child and also the new feelings it brings with being a family. I love watching our son grow and change and enjoy the funny things he does . . . I enjoy sharing this with my partner.*
>
> Sarah, 35, *mother of one child aged one*

This mother's comments reflect a common reply to this question – that motherhood had given them a new, rewarding relationship with another person, had created a family and added a new and positive dimension to her relationship with her partner. Susan Bram in her study of parents, childless and delaying couples found that these affiliative advantages of parenthood were recognized by all groups.[19] Becoming a mother is also a basis for new friendships – as many women meet other new mothers at antenatal and postnatal groups. Some describe this experience as providing a sense of unity with other women.[3,10]

PERSONAL FULFILMENT AND ACHIEVEMENT

For some women becoming a mother is also an opportunity for self development or personal expression:

Being a mother has allowed me to 'do' childhood again . . . I can have fun, joke – be a kid too . . . it's a sense of freedom . . . I enjoy being involved in her busy life.
> Jenny, 34, mother of one child aged four

A sense of achievement is also obtained from being a mediator in the child's development.

[It is rewarding] when you listen to your child getting wiser and see a lovely nature and personality evolving . . . it is nice to take some credit.
> Elizabeth, 36, mother of one child aged four

Two fantastic, lovely children are rewarding for me – the cuddles, love, joy and seeing them develop and experience things. It is worth juggling my life and coming to terms with the negatives.
> Phillipa, 39, mother of two children aged three and four

GENETIC IMMORTALITY

For some men and women having a child provides a sense of continuity. In the Australian study a few parents described this in terms of '*carrying the family on*' or as '*contributing to the future*'. For most, this was described as an enjoyment of seeing characteristics of themselves or their partner in the child. Susan Bram reports that some of the couples she studied saw having a child as a source of power in this respect – '*having an impact on the world*'.[19]

In summary, the negatives of having children relate to the more tangible, functional aspects of life, particularly career and finance. There are also potential negative effects on lifestyle and relationships though many parents describe these as the positive aspects of parenthood. Becoming a parent is a major life event bringing about an irreversible change – *a rite of passage*. Though their timing varies the majority of women opt for this change; a minority do not.

༆

Choosing a childfree life

Given the biological, psychological and social pressures which direct people toward having children it could be argued that there is relatively little choice but to become a parent. To choose to be childfree is certainly to go against the flow.

> Those who wish to remain childless are often seen as maladjusted, unfulfilled, immoral, or selfish and their freedom is sometimes the source of jealous annoyance to others.[23]

However, increasingly women are choosing to be childfree. A Canadian study reported that in 1979 five to seven per cent of all married couples had chosen not to have children and of these a third had made this decision before marriage.[24] In Gina Johnson's study of British women only two per cent of the total 12 per cent of women without children were involuntarily childless – for the majority it was a conscious choice.[25]

What is it that distinguishes this group from the majority whose preference is to have children? Two separate studies which have compared mothers, those intending to have children but delaying, and childfree individuals, suggest that those who are childfree are distinctly different from those who delay parenthood.[19,26,27] The delaying group hold values more akin to those who are already parents. The difference is in priorities and life values. While parents, delayers and childfree individuals all are able to describe advantages of having children, those in the childfree group give lower priority to these. Janet Reading and Ellen Amatea found that childfree women perceive the motivations for child-bearing as primarily selfish – for self-satisfaction – while those who have children define their motivations as altruistic – directing their love to others.[28]

Childfree women derive satisfaction from alternative sources. Voluntarily childless women are typically high achievers with demanding careers and, perhaps most importantly, describe their work as exciting and a source of great personal satisfaction.[19,24]

For these women to have a child is too great a sacrifice. The childfree place a much greater value on work/career than other women – including career women who delay parenthood. Susan Bram reports that in her sample of voluntarily childless women some found work more important not only than children but, for a large percentage, their marriage also. A subset of the childfree women in this study, however, derived their personal satisfaction from creativity and leisure pursuits rather than career.[19]

Psychological differences have been found between those who opt for a childfree life and those who choose parenthood. They place greater emphasis on autonomy and independence.[24,29] This is reflected in their style of marriage which has been found to be typically more egalitarian (less defined sex roles) and to allow greater independence. Janet Reading and Ellen Amatea report that women who choose to be childfree identify more with their fathers.[28] It is perhaps not surprising that those who choose to remain childfree are autonomous individuals who are satisfied with their existing career and lifestyle. This is a less conventional option – in many ways a brave one. The choice to become a mother is for many also a brave decision.

ᨠ
Choosing to have a child later

In an era where extended families are no longer the norm and experience of children less readily available, the decision to have a child is a leap into the unknown. For those who have developed busy autonomous lives centred around a career, travel and personal pursuits, the decision to have a child represents a major change. It marks an entry into a completely different world. For women who have delayed parenthood this is particularly likely to be so:

> *At my age it was a case of now or never . . . but it felt like jumping off the edge of a cliff.*
>
> Sandra, 36

I decided I had to take the plunge. My excuses had run out – career, holidays, money, etc.

Vivienne, 32

For other women who have delayed child-bearing this decision comes as a natural step once other achievements have been made:

My husband and I had reached a comfortable plateau in our relationship. I felt I could cope better with the changes a child would bring, though I had no idea really what these changes would be.

Grace, 35

A wide range of factors influence when this decision is made. For some, it is not so much a decision but a result of circumstance. The next section looks at the factors that affect the timing of parenthood – both planned and unplanned.

༂

Decisions about the timing of parenthood

Chance and choice: why women have babies when they do

Why do women have babies when they do? The reasons for any one pregnancy are likely to be complex with many contributing factors, both conscious and sub-conscious. It is not possible here to cover all of the possible factors that influence the timing of pregnancy. However, there are two major themes that emerge in all studies of the timing of motherhood and in women's personal accounts. The first is the issue of planning – whether a pregnancy resulted as a conscious choice or contraception failure. The second is the issue of wanting – whether a pregnancy results from a positive desire to have a child and whether it is received positively.

PLANNED BABIES?

It has been argued that the widespread knowledge about and availability of contraceptive technology in the developed world enables women to prevent unwanted pregnancies in most cases.[30,31] Most technological contraceptive methods have been found to have success rates exceeding 90 per cent.[31] These figures, however, contrast markedly with those for unplanned pregnancies. One study reports that only half of the annual pregnancies in the United States are 'intended'.[32] Studies in the United Kingdom document similar figures. Two studies conducted in British antenatal clinics found that approximately half of all pregnancies were unplanned.[33,34] Alison While in a study of Health Visitor records and unpublished figures from the Children of the Nineties study indicate that a third of all pregnancies which proceed to live births are unplanned.[35,36] Though there is some variation between studies these figures all testify to a discrepancy between the possibility of planning a baby presented by contraceptive technology and the reality. They suggest that there is a substantial proportion of pregnancies which falls between the category of truly unplanned pregnancies, defined as contraception failure, and planned pregnancies. These pregnancies have resulted from some element of risk-taking and are perhaps best termed 'unintended' or 'less intended' pregnancies. Three examples from the Australian Timing of Motherhood study are typical:[9]

My first pregnancy was an accident, but the best mistake I ever made. My second was slightly more planned and just as enjoyable. I think if you are in a happy stable relationship timing doesn't matter.

Joanne, 21 at first birth

Although my pregnancy was an accident I would not have allowed such a situation to arise if I had not been in a stable, long-term relationship.

Sue, 23 at first birth

I didn't exactly plan my pregnancy . . . becoming pregnant saved me from having to make a decision.

Louise, 30 at first birth

Several studies have found that the number of such unintended pregnancies varies with age. Alison While reports that in her study the number of planned pregnancies increased significantly with maternal age.[35] The Australian Timing of Motherhood study reports a similar finding.[9] In this study mothers were asked to rate how planned their pregnancies were on a five-point rating scale. Significant differences between late and early timing mothers were found with late timing mothers more likely to have a very planned pregnancy and younger mothers a pregnancy which was definitely not planned. In this study the range of later timing mothers was from 30 to 42 years with the majority in the range 33 to 38 years. A study of women who had babies over the age of 40 found that unplanned pregnancies were high amongst women in this group.[37,38] It is likely that the cause of unplanned pregnancy for these women is different from that in women younger than forty with misguided beliefs about their own fertility playing a greater role in the 40-plus group.[37,38,39] In both age groups, however, covert and subconscious motives for having a child are also likely to play a role.

Table 3.1. Planning of pregnancy for early, (under 25), average (25–29) and late (30 or more) timing mothers in the Australian Timing of Motherhood study

Timing	Early (n=50) %	Average (n=30) %	Late (n=60) %
Very planned	33	66	64
Planned	4	15	25
Only moderately	13	3	4
Not really	18	7	2
Definitely not	32	9	5

WANTED BABIES?

The terms unplanned and unwanted are often used as if they were synonymous. However, many unplanned pregnancies become wanted just as planned and intended pregnancies become unwanted. Also the term 'unwanted' does not describe the ambivalence felt by many women on finding themselves unexpectedly pregnant.[1]

Maureen Freely & Celia Pyper

The timing of motherhood is not determined simply by the use or failure to use contraception. Conceiving and having a child is an intensely personal and emotional experience and underlying rational decisions and behaviours about fertility are a maze of individual motives, feelings and circumstance. Maureen Freely and Celia Pyper in their book *Pandora's Clock* draw upon the mythical Pandora's box to capture the mystical and uncontained nature of fertility decisions.[1] They suggest that underlying many ostensibly unplanned pregnancies is a logic of unspoken desires. Many pregnancies are conceived where the circumstances are not objectively ideal, yet a child is desired. Social norms may dictate that pregnancy is not appropriate at a given time: for example because a women is young, unmarried or at the wrong stage of career, but the desire may still be present. In these ambivalent circumstances there is a higher likelihood of risk-taking with contraception. Similarly, when one partner in a couple has a desire to have a child before another the motivation for contraceptive vigilance by that partner may drop. An unintended pregnancy in both these circumstances will bring about a resolution of the conflict between what 'should' be done and the desire to have a child by removing the responsibility of choice.

> *. . . It's the pressure of age . . . I wish I had 10 more years left to decide . . . it's such a big decision . . . I've talked to my doctor about using more 'dangerous' contraceptive methods – barrier methods – so there is scope for an accident. If I had an accident the decision would be made for me. It is too big a decision to make.*
>
> *Lindsey, 38, currently without children*

> *I am glad I had an accident. I wouldn't like to be faced with the decision to have children like you are – it's too big a decision to make.*
>
> *Letter to one of the authors, then aged 32, from her sister who conceived her first child unintentionally 12 years previously at the age of 21*

Emotions broadly termed as wanting a child not only explain the timing of unintended pregnancies, but would appear to be the major contributing factor to the timing of most pregnancies. In the Australian Timing of Motherhood study *'feeling emotionally ready'* was outstandingly the most influential determinant of the timing of pregnancy whether planned or unplanned and whether to a younger mother or an older mother.[9] There were differences in how the desire for a child was experienced, however. For younger mothers this was more commonly described as either a destiny or instinct, whereas for older mothers the feeling of readiness was more commonly described as something that had been acquired with time – either emotional maturity or emotional stability that had followed achievement of other life goals.

> *I felt ready to be a mother having done so much in life already. Feeling secure . . . and more mature – it helps a lot with finding the balance between being a mother and retaining self-identity.*
>
> *Phillipa, 39, aged 35 at first birth*

> *I was feeling content – satisfied with my career achievements, travel experiences and relationship – I was ready to have a child.*
>
> *Serena, 33 at first birth*

For those women who experience fertility problems wanting a child is not so much the key to the timing of having a baby but it is perhaps the overriding motivation to which we can attribute their persistence despite often physically and emotionally taxing fertility treatments:

> *Sometimes I feel like I am on a treadmill of treatment that is for the doctor's benefit rather than mine.*
>
> *Jane, awaiting egg donation*

Design and circumstance: why do women become mothers later?

PART OF THE PLAN: CHOOSING TO HAVE A FIRST BABY AFTER 35

Why do women choose to have a first child later? One possibility is that women who have children later are those who intended to be childfree but changed their mind 'at the last minute'. Research studies suggest that the decision of whether or not to have a child at all is made at a much earlier life stage and that those who choose to be childfree are likely to adhere to this decision. Later timing women, on the other hand, are likely to have had a long term intention to become a mother but have delayed.[19,27]

Because a significant proportion of women who voluntarily delay motherhood have a high level of education and established careers it is often assumed that career considerations are the overriding explanation for delayed parenthood. Certainly career plays a role. Undertaking further education delays entry into the adult world of working and earning and therefore places practical constraints upon the decision to become a parent. Some careers such as medicine have lengthy postgraduate training which further extends these constraints.[40] Studies which have directly questioned women about their motives for delay, however, portray a far more complex picture.

Benjamin and Rachel Schlesinger, in their review of a range of studies on delayed parenthood, report that while career is a consistent theme, the need for financial and emotional security were equally common reasons cited for delay.[41] Julia Berryman and Kate Windridge's study of women having children over 40 reports that finance is more important than career as a factor in timing while Karen Thorpe and Jana Cinnamon's study of Australian women found that career was ranked below factors associated with emotional security.[9] Maxine Soloway and Rebbecca Smith suggest that family messages about life priorities and timing of parenthood play an important part in the decision to delay parenting.[8] Their in-depth study of 15 couples who had delayed parenting until their mid-thirties indicated that family values dictated that their twenties were a time for education and establishment of a career identity, financial security and relationship with a partner. This study did not have a comparison group of early timing parents but other studies have suggested that family values may play a role in influencing early timing as well. Harriet Presser, for example, reports that the role model provided by a woman's mother is a key factor:[42] she found that the single greatest predictor of early timing motherhood was early timing by the woman's own mother.

What factors influence women delaying motherhood to eventually have a child? Maxine Soloway and Rebecca Smith suggest that a re-evaluation of the values which underly the delay occur after thirty.[8] The major trigger for this re-evaluation was the pressure of the biological time clock. The pressure of age and the finite duration of female fertility are key elements in the timing of later, planned pregnancies. The crisis of age is the catalyst for the decision to accept some of the negative aspects of parenthood and 'take the plunge' into the relatively unknown world of parenthood.

At what age does this crisis of the biological clock occur? The first psychological age barrier is 30. For many people turning 30 is a significant life event but for women who have not yet had children it can be particularly poignant. Though the age at which women are having children is increasing (*see Chapter 2*) the perceptions of women are that 30 is later than average and outside the norm. Perhaps more importantly, 30 is the age at which women begin to perceive that age is a risk to the health of mother and baby and a threat to fertility. Responses from women in the Australian Timing of Motherhood study clearly portray this:[9]

I didn't want to start much later for reasons of medical risk and I didn't want to be an elderly parent.

Clare, 29 at first birth

The ideal time to have a child is between 25 and 29 when you are not too old. If you decide to have children and then find you have problems, it gives you time to get through the red tape of adoption or to have fertility treatment.

Elise, 27 at first birth

The view that motherhood after 30 is somewhat different and associated with risk is also conveyed in popular literature and medical writing which until recently have used the age 30 as the point at which a pregnant woman is termed an 'elderly primigravida'.

More recently, the medical definition of later motherhood has adopted 35 as the age at which mothers are defined as an exceptional medical group – reflecting a recognition of the general population trend to delaying motherhood and the low 'risk' for the new population of later mothers having children in their early thirties (*see Chapter 4*). In reports and studies of women's views about the timing of motherhood, 30 is overwhelmingly the age identified as the turning point at which women feel pressure to become a mother, however. For those who intend to have children but have not done so 35 is the next important landmark, however. There is an increasing awareness that 35 is the medical definition of age-associated risk to pregnancy because this is the age at which additional screening procedures, CVS and amniocentesis, are made available on the basis of age alone. These are described in Chapters 5 and 6. Although risks are lower than for those who remain childfree, recent reports have also publicized a potentially increased risk of breast cancer to women having a first child over 35 – again a signal of this age as critical in decision making about the timing of motherhood (*see Chapter 5 for a detailed discussion of medical risk*).[43,44,45]

In the Australian Timing of Motherhood study when asked about the best age to have children many women recognized that after 35 there are advantages of maturity and security but questioned the ability of women at this age to cope with a young child because they perceived they would not have enough energy.[9] Of the sample who had actually had their children after 35 energy levels were indeed an issue with some questioning whether parenthood would have been less tiring at an earlier age. The only actual evidence about this comes from the Leicester Motherhood Project which found that there was not, in fact, a difference between reports of tiredness between younger and older mothers 16 to 17 weeks after the birth.[46] It is possible that differences occur later in parenthood but it is more probable that motherhood is a tiring occupation regardless of age. However, older mothers are more likely to blame age for feeling this way. Interestingly, in the Australian Timing of Motherhood study the social acceptability of being a parent after 35 was not raised as an issue in choice of best age for motherhood.[9]

In summary, then, career, finance, personal identity and security are the key factors which have been given as reasons for delaying first-time motherhood and these are influenced by family values. The pressure of the biological clock is the key factor in proceeding to have a child: this pressure is often felt at 30 and becomes more critical at 35 when there is a greater perception of medical risk and concern about coping with the energy demands of motherhood.

FORCE OF CIRCUMSTANCE: UNINTENDED DELAY

For some women circumstances conspire to determine the time at which they first have children. Two primary reasons for this are the experience of fertility problems and the delay in finding an appropriate partner.

Fertility problems can result in substantial postponement of parenthood from the chosen age of timing. The normal range of time for conception is up to 12 months so that quite some time is likely to be taken before identifying that a problem exists. For women who conceive but experience miscarriage, this is again the case. Investigations are not usually undertaken unless a woman has experienced three consecutive miscarriages. Once a problem has been identified there may be further delays before investigations of both partners are undertaken. Waiting times for treatment and success rates for different treatments vary and it is possible that many years may pass before a successful pregnancy is achieved. For women waiting for egg donation, for example, the wait for a donor can be very long and difficult.[7] The financial and emotional burden of treatment may mean that women do not stay on a programme continually and this may be a further source of delay. Given these circumstances it is not surprising that women experiencing fertility problems who through choice would have timed motherhood at late twenties or early thirties actually become mothers after 35.

While many women by their late twenties have established a partnership there are, of course, many who are single in their thirties. Most of these women are unlikely to take the option of single motherhood but rather delay parenthood until they are established in a relationship:

When I met my husband, we agreed that we would try for a family as soon as we could. Had we met when we were younger I believe we would still have done this . . . so it was not a case of choosing but circumstance.

Anne, 35 at first birth

There was no timing involved: if I had met my partner three years earlier I would have become a mother three years earlier.

Ellen, 36 at first birth

For some women it is not finding a partner but the attitude of the partner which is the reason for delay. The sense of urgency of the biological clock ticking away is not felt by some partners, particularly if they are younger:

My husband is five years younger than I am so we had to balance my biological clock with his youthfulness.

Helene, 35 at first birth

࿔

Decisions about family size and spacing

Age undoubtedly affects decisions about the number of children a woman will have and spacing between pregnancies. Many women who plan their first child in their early thirties will have subsequent children beyond the age of 35.

ONLY CHILDREN

The average family has two or three children and studies have shown that younger women's expectations are that they will have more than one child. Concern about having an only child, particularly about the possibility of this adversely affecting the child, is a concern often voiced by mothers. For those who have had their first child later it may become a greater issue. The pressure of time and the perceived risks of later pregnancy are weighed against guilt and concern about having only one child. For those who have conceived as a result of fertility treatment the issue of stress is a greater one. Conceiving subsequent pregnancies may again require such technological assistance and the physical, emotional and financial cost of further treatment must be weighed against the issue of the only child (*see Chapter 10 for further discussion*).

MULTIPLE BIRTH

One special issue which is particularly relevant to women with fertility problems is that of multiple birth. Treatment for fertility carries with it a risk of multiple birth. All multiple births, but particularly higher order multiple births (three or more) carry a high risk of abnormality and obstetric complication and the emotional and financial costs of care after the birth are high.[47] Here the decision is between the possibility of no child and more than one at once. Most women in these circumstances opt for fertility treatment in the belief that they will have two children at most. IVF programmes limit the number of implanted embryos to three and so the likelihood of higher order multiple birth is reduced. With drug treatments, however, there is less control. In some higher order multiple pregnancies selective reduction of the number of babies is carried out to give the remaining babies a greater chance of survival and health. This procedure is not without risk and may result in the total loss of a much wanted pregnancy. The devastating effect of losing a pregnancy in this case is compounded by the guilt of playing an active part in this loss.

Being pregnant is like knitting – each day is another stitch of fantasy: what the baby will be like, what it will look like. Then you lose it and have to go back and laboriously unpick up all these stitches. It was about a year before I could think of having a baby in my arms without crying.[47]

Anna, who lost her pregnancy following selective feticide

The issue of selective termination raises difficult ethical issues for parents and medical staff alike.[48]

'PACKING THEM IN': CLOSE SPACING

A decision to have further children may mean a decision to have more closely spaced children because of the perceived pressures of time. This may make parenting more pressured and stressful. A study by Karen Thorpe and colleagues has found that closer spacing of children is more stressful and may have an adverse effect on the emotional well-being of the mother.[49]

Some women also express concern that closer spacing of children might adversely affect their physical well-being. There is evidence that a very short inter-pregnancy interval (less than four months) increases risks of foetal and infant death but not of adverse effects on the health of the mother.[50] Importantly, no differences in reported health during pregnancy or the post-partum have been found from women of different ages.[9] Recovery is more likely to relate to individual fitness and number of children than age.[50] Despite this finding some women who start to have children later hold a belief that it will take longer for their older bodies to recover from pregnancy and childbirth and express concern about the impact of closer spacing:

I would like to have another baby but my body is only just feeling like it's mine again. So if you plan to postpone pregnancy until your forties it is worth considering that you may have less time to have a second child.[51]

Kitty, 43 at first birth

'SECOND FAMILIES': HAVING ANOTHER CHILD AFTER A LONG TIME

There are a number of circumstances which lead women to consider having children a long time after previous children. The new child or children are like second families. A new relationship may be one reason for this family pattern. In these circumstances concern about the reaction of existing children and former partner may be an issue. There is evidence that a second family may adversely affect a woman's relationship with her former spouse and, as a consequence, have an impact on the children's relationship also, but a new baby may add a positive dimension to the new relationship.

It is not uncommon for second families to occur for the same couple.

> *Simon was an accident . . . at 37 with my children all safely at school I hadn't intended to have more. Now I have got him I think I will have another. I do not want him to be like an only child. It will be like two families and the girls are so good with him it makes it much easier.*
>
> Geraldine, 37, *mother of two girls aged eleven and nine and a son aged six months*

Often in this circumstance the pregnancy is less intended but, as was the case for Geraldine, and Betty in Chapter 1, the new child is eventually seen as a positive outcome.

In second families whether for an existing or new relationship the decisions about family size and spacing are the same as those of first-timers but arise for a second time.

GOING FOR A THIRD OR MORE?

For some women starting a family later puts constraints on the size of the family they will have. Whether to have further children, typically a third child, becomes an issue because this child is likely to be born to a woman who is in her late thirties or early forties. In this context, too, concerns about medical risk and energy levels are commonly raised:

> *We are trying to decide whether to have a third but are thinking that we may be a little elderly. We like the idea of romping with our children.*
>
> Catherine, 36, mother of two

For parents who have all children of the same sex the desire to have a child of the opposite sex may be a key issue.

> *I've always wanted a daughter . . . if I knew I would have a girl I'd definitely go for a third but it is a gamble isn't it? Pregnancy doesn't get easier.*
>
> Rosemary, 36, mother of two boys

Studies on this issue covering a range of cultures, including Britain and the US, have found that the majority of men and women have a preference for a boy child. According to a large study by Lois Hoffman couples are more likely to continue to have children if they have only girls. They will have more children than they originally planned in order to fulfill their desire for a son.[52]

Clearly there are many decisions about motherhood which lead a woman to become a mother after 35. The reasons for later motherhood, whether voluntarily or involuntarily, first-time or last, are seldom simple. The stereotypic notions of single-minded career women squeezing a child in, or of a woman with long-term fertility problems miraculously having a baby later, are oversimplistic. The range of women who become mothers after 35 and the circumstances in which this comes about is diverse: As Pamela Daniels and Kathy Weingarten put it:[53]

> The timing of mid-life parenthood may be not so much the outcome of programmatic planning as the culmination of a long process of deferral in which intention and circumstances, desire and delay, are threaded unevenly in and around each other.[53]

༑ 4 ༑

'Trying' for a Baby after 35:
Getting and Staying Pregnant

By 35 only half of all women can conceive; this figure is reduced
to 3–4% by age 44.[1]

James Brew, obstetrician and gynaecologist, 1982

In a natural population, when women marry in their late 30s or
early 40s, perhaps one-third to one-half of couples will remain
involuntarily childless.[2]

Paul Gindoff and Raphael Jewelewicz,
both obstetricians and gynaecologists, 1986

For anyone wishing to become pregnant after 35 these comments
may seem surprising, even shocking. Fortunately it is likely that
the more pessimistic of these views does not accurately reflect the
average woman's chances of having a baby after 35 today. Such
assertions are misleading and may well be influenced by *fertility
statistics* – the number of babies actually born to women – rather
than the true potential to bear children. As we pointed out in
Chapter 2, fertility statistics only reveal what women *do* and not
what they *could* do. In a world where women control their fertility
estimating women's potential to bear children is not easy.

This chapter addresses issues surrounding getting pregnant
and staying pregnant. We discuss a woman's potential to bear
children in relation to her age and the factors that may hinder
conception. In addition assisted conception is considered, as are
the chances of miscarriage once conception is achieved.

ॐ
A woman's potential to bear a baby

There is little consensus amongst the 'experts' on the extent of the decline in fertility with age and the quotations at the start of this chapter represent only one extreme of the range of opinions available. Other researchers, including the authors of this book, believe that there is evidence to suggest that women's chances of having a baby after 35 are still much better than 50 percent and we shall go on to consider the evidence for a more gradual decline in fertility.

In his book on pregnancy Gordon Bourne suggests that about three quarters of women between 36 and 40 who wish to become pregnant will do so, providing that they have intercourse at the rate of three or more times a week.[3] Amongst the most fertile (i.e. the most prolific) human population known, the Hutterites, the probability of having a live birth at a given age does show a decline as women get older but the likelihood of having a baby is much greater than the introductory comments suggest.[4] The peak age for having babies was found to be the twentieth year of life, in the study reported in 1953, when just over 60 per cent of all married women of that age had a live birth. At the age of 35 the proportion of married women having a baby fell to just over 45 per cent in that year. This shows a decline compared with the peak age (taken as 100 per cent) to 74.1 per cent for *annual* live births amongst married women. This proportion drops to approximately 50 per cent at age 40 when just under one third (32 per cent) of married women were reported to give birth in their fortieth year.

Whilst these figures are not exactly comparable with other studies they suggest that fertility is still high because at the age of 40, on average, a woman could still expect at least one more live birth (*see Table 2.3 in Chapter 2*). The figures reported for the Hutterites show annual births by age, but as fertility declines the gaps between babies may increase. Nevertheless the likelihood of having another baby at some stage was still very real for Hutterite women at 40, suggesting that the majority of the population is still 'at risk' of pregnancy.

Estimates of sterility by age in the Hutterites have been calculated by Christopher Tietze[5] who notes that sterility in couples where the woman is aged 34 years is 11 per cent, at 39 years is 33 per cent and at 44 years is 87 per cent. It should be noted that the extents to which male infertility and reduction of rates of intercourse influence these figures are unknown but will undoubtedly play a part. From this data it appears that at 39 two thirds of women have the potential to bear children.

∿

Fertility in past times

Louis Henry reports some interesting statistics from historical data.[6] Taking fertility to be at a maximum level at 20–24 years, in women married at 20, he produced figures from 13 populations not practising birth control, which indicate that fertility declines to 68.7 per cent at 35–39 years and to 5 per cent at 45–49 years. Henry's fertility data is taken from a wide range of populations such as the 'Bourgeoisie, of Geneva, wives of men born between 1600 and 1649', 'marriages from 1945–1946 in Hindu villages of Bengal', 'Crulai, Normandy, marriages from 1674–1742'. Figures for the Hutterites are also included.

His figure for absolute sterility is approximately three per cent for women aged 20 (*see Tables 4.1 and 4.2*) which increases to 16 per cent for married women aged 35, and 31 per cent at 40 – this latter data is taken from European populations. Thus this historical data, taken from populations where diet and health may have been considerably poorer than today, shows that fertility was still high up to the age of 40. The most positive information on the probability of conception – *fecundability* as it is called – has come from populations not practising birth control. Since most present day populations practise birth control much of the historical data available is not comparable with Western populations of today where, in general, women are better fed, healthier and longer lived than their historical counterparts. As was pointed out in Chapter 2 only the Hutterite data, published in the 1950s, comes close to resembling, in these terms, women in the Western world today.

Table 4.1. Natural fertility: the average of age-specific fertility rates for 13 populations not practising birth control

	20–24 years	25–29 years	30–34 years	35–39 years	40–44 years	45–49 years
Average	100*	93.5	85.3	68.7	34.9	5

* Where fertility is assumed to be at its maximum for any given populations.
Source: Henry's data, 1961[6]

Table 4.2 Age-specific Percentages of Sterility in Married Women

Population	20 years	25 years	30 years	35 years	40 years
Average (European populations)	3	6	10	16	31

Source: Henry's data, 1961[6].

One other source of information on fecundability comes from statistics on the success of artificial insemination for women of different ages. These data have advantages over those from natural populations in that they are not confounded by the possible impact of male infertility, and the reduction of frequency of intercourse, associated with increasing age and length of marriage.

乃

Fertility today

Artificial insemination by donor (AID) is a method of achieving a pregnancy which is generally sought when a woman's partner is subfertile or infertile, or occasionally by single women or lesbian couples wishing to become pregnant.

Table 4.3. Success of AID by age of women

Age in years	Success rate (%)
<25	73
26–30	74.1
31–35	61.5
>35	53.6

Source: Schwartz & Mayaux, 1982[7].

A major study of AID in France recorded the success rate of 2193 women of a variety of different ages.[7] Table 4.3 shows their success rates. At age 25, 73 per cent of women conceived, dropping to 53.6 per cent at 35-plus. The participants in this study are presumed to have no gynaecological disease and thus this procedure should reveal the *natural decline* in fertility with age.

Comparing these results with natural populations the success rate appears to be rather low. For example, other research in the US showed that 63 per cent of women between the ages of 35 and 39 were fecund in a 1965 study.[8] Why does this discrepancy occur?

Richard Gosden points out that natural insemination is often twice as successful as artificial insemination – in terms of the number of conceptions achieved per woman per month.[9] In the French study only 0.1 successful conceptions were obtained per woman per month whereas success may reach 0.4–0.5 in optimally fertile couples when intercourse occurs daily. Sperm are damaged during the freezing and thawing required for AID, and the procedure itself may be carried out at a time in the cycle when the fertile period is missed. In addition to this, the stress on couples undertaking the procedure should not be underestimated. The procedure is usually carried out in secret because couples often do not wish others to know that the fertility of the male partner is in question. This aspect of the procedure can put a considerable strain on individuals receiving AID and it may play a role in reducing the success rate.

Thus although AID would seem to be the best method of assessing decline in fertility with age (since rates of intercourse and male problems do not influence the results), in reality natural insemination is much more successful. At over 35, a 63 per cent success rate is still likely to be an underestimate, for the reasons already stated.

ॐ

Women's expectations about getting pregnant after 35

In the Leicester Motherhood Project all the participants were asked about their feelings on trying to become pregnant.[10] Half our sample was aged 35 or over at the time of the first interview early in their pregnancy, and these are some of the comments from the first-time mothers.

> *We'd given up . . . accepted our life as it was.*
>
> *Elaine*

> *I assumed I was too old.*
>
> *Marie*

> *We had had treatment for 12 years – but never let it take over – always managed to laugh about it. Tried to plan life round coping without pregnancy.*
>
> *Ruth*

This selection of comments, from first-time mothers, suggests clearly that many have a low expectation of pregnancy by the time they achieved their 35-plus pregnancy.

Our sample targeted all first-time 35-plus mothers at the largest hospital in Leicestershire, and these comments are typical of those who volunteered to take part. A number of these women had been trying to become pregnant for some years so their pessimism is not too surprising.

In our study of 40-plus mothers more than half the target babies of this study, born on or after their mother's fortieth birthday, were unplanned and 40 per cent of the first-time mothers had sought fertility advice prior to the pregnancy.[11] Mothers were not asked about their feelings about trying to become pregnant but it is of interest that 60 per cent, when asked whether they always assumed they would have children answered that they assumed they would not. Clearly expectations about the later pregnancy were low. This feeling is reflected in another survey of British women which reported that few childless women aged between 40 and 44 believe that they could conceive. Only five per cent of childless women thought that they could, whereas a third of women who have a child already think they could have another one at this age.[12]

ↄ

The time taken to conceive

Of course the decline in fertility indicated by the above figures gives no clues to the time taken to conceive and for the woman aged 35 or over this is probably what she is really interested in. The questions 'Will I get pregnant?' and 'How long will it take?' are what most women who are hoping to have a baby, want to know when they start 'trying'.

A study of women undergoing artificial insemination found that on average conception in women aged over 35 took over 12 months whereas the average time for those aged 31–35 years was seven months, and for those under 30 it was six months.[7]

Returning again to the most fertile women, Richard Gosden notes that the intervals between pregnancies for Hutterite women was:[9] 'surprisingly constant throughout reproductive life, apart from substantially longer intervals between the final two pregnancies'. Approximately a third of the population of married Hutterite women had a baby each year and this rate only dropped to a fifth amongst women aged 40–44 years. Of course the rate of intercourse, male infertility and the duration of breast-feeding are all factors that will influence these figures.

Other studies of more modern populations show that at 35 or so it is not unusual for women to have to wait a year or more to conceive. Ann Cartwright found, in her sample of women aged 35 and over, that of those who became pregnant, 40 per cent achieved a pregnancy within 6 months, but 47 per cent took two years or longer; of the remaining 13 per cent, 11 per cent took 6 months to a year and 2 per cent took 1–2 years.[13] In this study it was noted that length of marriage was correlated to time taken to conceive – longer marriages being linked to longer times to achieve conception and also to lower frequencies for intercourse.

In the Leicester Motherhood Project the time taken to conceive was under six months for the majority of women who were 'trying' to become pregnant (*see Table 4.4*) but over a quarter of first-time mothers of 35-plus took longer than two years to conceive their first-born.[10]

Table 4.4. Time taken to conceive, showing percentages of women by time (in months), in older and younger mothers 'trying' for a baby

Age groups and parity* of women	Time taken to conceive			
	0–6	7–12	13–24	24+
35+ primiparous	66.7	–	5.6	27.7
35+ multiparous	77.7	5.6	11.1	5.6
20–29 primiparous	82.6	–	8.7	8.7
20–29 multiparous	88.2	5.9	–	5.9

* Parity: primiparous mothers are first-time mothers, multiparous mothers are those with one or more previous children.
Source: Leicester Motherhood Project[10]

In the British study of 40-plus mothers the time taken to conceive was much higher than the above figures suggest.[11] The mean for first-time 40-plus mothers was nearly four years (i.e. 47.58 months) whereas for those with one or more previous children it was just over one year (i.e. 12.70 months). Of interest here was that women with previous children did not take significantly longer to conceive their 40-plus baby than they did for their first-born child which was born much earlier at an average age of 26.

To sum up, the 35-plus mother should not be surprised if conception takes some time – a year or two may not be unusual. Women concerned that there may be possible problems may wish to consult their doctor well within a year. In addition to this women should be aware that a number of factors concerned with lifestyle are now well known in influencing the likelihood of conception and we shall consider these next.

꒜

Other factors influencing the likelihood of conception

Body weight

One of the factors influencing the timing of the first menstrual period is a girl's weight. In Chapter 2 it was noted that the age of menarche has declined over the last century and one of the factors affecting this has been improved nutrition – girls are simply bigger than they used to be for any given age. The onset of menstruation seems to be linked to the requirement for a minimum level of stored fat (i.e. there may be a critical body weight for the onset of menstruation for a particular type of physique).[14] To put it simply the body is not ready to make babies unless it has some reserves of fat. Children who are short and stocky tend to achieve this weight sooner and mature earlier than those who are slimmer and taller.[15] For women, the amount of stored fat is also important; those who are excessively thin, who suffer from anorexia nervosa, or indeed athletes who train to increase muscle and reduce fat, are all likely to suppress ovulation and hence their capacity to have babies. Again there may be a critical weight necessary for the maintenance of menstrual cycles which is probably somewhat higher than that triggering onset at puberty.

Thus women who are overly concerned about a 'model' figure may jeopardize their chances of conception. A woman wishing to become pregnant should have a good diet and maintain at least an average body weight for her height – therefore slimming is unwise in those wishing to become pregnant.

On the other side of the coin it must also be emphasized that fatness also has an impact. In an article entitled 'Fat and female fecundity' Boukje Zaadstra and colleagues describe a study of 500 women receiving artificial insemination.[16] They found that the waist-hip ratio seemed to be an indicator of likely conception rates. The most common size of women in their sample was a waist-hip ratio of 0.75–0.80 (i.e. their waist was three quarters the size of their hips or a little bigger) but the highest proportion of women becoming pregnant was in the group having a ratio of less than 0.7. Sixty-three per cent of women became pregnant in this latter group, over 12 insemination cycles, and, as the ratio increased, the proportion fell to 32 per cent becoming pregnant amongst those with a ratio that was equal to, or bigger than 0.85. They summed up their research by saying that pear-shaped women have less difficulty in becoming pregnant than apple-shaped (big-waisted) women.

Breastfeeding

Although women today are warned not to rely on breastfeeding as a preventive to a further pregnancy, by the same token women wishing to become pregnant again, quickly, may also need to consider carefully how long they should continue to breastfeed their current baby. It is widely recognised that lactation limits the likelihood of conception:

> Throughout the world as a whole, more births are prevented by lactation than all other forms of contraception put together.[14]

Indeed in earlier times when diets may have been at marginal levels only, ovulation would be suppressed in the breastfeeding mother. This applies equally to the poor in underdeveloped countries today. Robert May has noted that women in earlier times were likely to have nursed their children for much longer periods than is common today.[17] Breastfeeding children for three or four years would not have been unusual and would lead to a natural spacing between children of about five years. There is a tendency for us today to assume that, prior to the occurrence of effective contraceptive techniques, a woman in much earlier times once married, or in a relationship, would continue to have children very frequently throughout her reproductive life. However, the more limited diet combined with lactation would be a crucial factor in preventing ovulation and thus increasing the interval between births.

The suppression of ovulation during breastfeeding is not only linked to diets at a marginal level; the frequency of sucking by the infant also plays a role. Research indicates that higher frequency sucking such as is often found in women feeding on demand, may produce 'lactational amenorrhoea'.[18] It is said that neural impulses from the teat affect hormonal balances and babies fed at a few scheduled times each day, rather than those fed on demand, therefore produce a lower frequency of the sucking stimulus. This lower frequency may be insufficient to suppress ovulation in a well fed mother. Thus women feeding on demand, even if on a more than adequate diet, may be suppressing ovulation and hence reducing their chances of a further baby.

The significance of these two factors may be minimal for younger mothers wishing to add to their families but for the older woman, approaching the end of her reproductive life, it may be necessary to balance the wish to breastfeed against the wish for further pregnancy. This is especially so for those planning to breastfeed for a long period.

Smoking

The link between smoking and pregnancy outcome is well documented as are its effects on the unborn child during pregnancy.[19]

Smoking increases the risk of miscarriage, premature birth and leads to a baby that is 'small for dates' – this means that the baby is not as big as is expected for a given number of weeks gestation. Smoking has the effect of making the placenta function less well thus it is a major hazard to pregnancy.

Less well known is the effect of smoking on the ability to conceive and this is our chief concern in this chapter. Women who smoke increase conception delay and this is more marked in older women.[20] A major population study – that is a study of all mothers, in a certain district (in this case the city of Tampere, Finland) – of 2198 women aged between 14 and 44, who reached mid-pregnancy, reported data from interviews regarding women's smoking habits, those of their husband or partner, and a range of other factors relevant to fecundity such as previous pregnancies, abortions and so on.[20] It was found that smoking not only affected conception rate, but its effects were more marked the *longer* the conception delay became. The deleterious effect of even light smoking became more significant as time taken to conceive increased.

Maternal smoking was not the only factor to influence conception. Paternal smoking also had an effect and amongst women who became successfully pregnant in 12 months, partner smoking also increased the risk of conception delay. Thus women wishing to become pregnant, especially older women, should not only give up smoking themselves, but should bear in mind that a partner who smokes may also jeopardize the rate at which they will conceive.

A variety of other studies have investigated this issue and found similar adverse effects of smoking. One study found that smokers were 3.4 times more likely to take *more than a year* to conceive than non-smokers, and decreasing fertility has been linked to an increasing number of cigarettes per day.[21]

However, one marginally positive effect of smoking has been noted; the mother who smokes is less likely to develop pre-eclampsia (one of the chief symptoms is raised blood pressure) but, if she does get pre-eclampsia, as Sheila Kitzinger points out, 'she gets it worse than a non-smoking mother and the outcome for the fetus is worse.'[19]

On balance, the message is simple: women wishing to become pregnant are advised not to smoke and the adverse effects of not taking this advice are greater for the older woman.

Coffee and cola

There is some controversy over the link between coffee drinking and the chances of conception. One study has reported that women who drank the equivalent of more than one cup of coffee per day were *half* as likely to conceive per cycle, whilst another much larger study of over 3000 women who had had babies found that conception took longest for those who drank four or more cups of coffee per day.[22]

Francine Grodstein and colleagues have tried to find out exactly what effect coffee, or more precisely caffeine, has on fertility.[23] They studied almost 5000 women, of whom over 1000 had primary infertility, and the remainder had given birth to at least one child. They found that amongst those with high levels of caffeine intake there was a significant risk of infertility due to tubal disease or endometriosis. Women who drank the approximate equivalent of more than two cups of coffee, or four cans of cola, per day (i.e. more than 7g of caffeine per month) showed a 1.5 fold increase in the risk of tubal infertility relative to those who drank less than half this amount. Increased risks for endometriosis were found for those consuming slightly less – about 5g of caffeine per month. The authors of this research note a number of possible limitations to their study but are persuaded that caffeine does require further careful investigation because they believe that there is now enough evidence to be concerned that it may have an adverse effect on the female reproductive system.

In 1980 the Food and Drug Administration in America suggested limiting caffeine use during pregnancy but this is not currently part of the standard recommendations issued by the American College of Obstetrics and Gynecology.[23] For brief details of other research into caffeine in pregnancy see Chapter 6.

Pre-conceptional counselling

Today it is common for those who are planning to start a family to have counselling concerning the ways in which they can improve their lifestyle and health to promote a healthy pregnancy and baby. It is not the intention of the authors to address the many issues which such courses might explore. Our purpose has been to point out several areas of particular relevance to women of 35 or older which might affect their chances of conception. Women wishing to have pre-conceptional counselling are advised to discuss this with their doctor.

৶

Assisted conception

For the woman who has done everything she can to increase her chances of a pregnancy but is 35 or more, an inability to conceive over some months may give rise to concern and worry. A visit to her doctor at this stage may reassure her that her chances are still good – because as we have noted it is not unusual for conception to take a year or so after 35. A woman over 35 may be investigated for infertility sooner than a young one, whilst a woman in her twenties may be asked to wait a year or more before beginning investigations. Although it may take longer for a woman over 35 to conceive, any delay in identifying a problem as she approaches her late thirties puts a delay into the system which she can ill afford.

Once investigations are begun a woman and her partner will both be involved. The man's fertility will probably be checked early on because this is a fairly straightforward procedure.[24] Samples of sperm (at least two) must be provided (by masturbation) and these will be assessed. If a problem is identified here then treatment, where possible, can be started. If a male problem is then excluded a wide range of investigations of the woman will continue. For most couples fertility problems will be due solely to the man in about one third of cases, solely to the woman in another third of cases, and the remainder may be due to shared problems. There is now a wide range of material available for couples to read (*see recommended reading*) for those with fertility problems but in this chapter we shall briefly consider some of the relatively new treatments that are available for women who cannot achieve conception naturally.

Test-tube babies: in-vitro fertilization

At one time, in the 1970s and earlier, a woman with blocked Fallopian tubes which could not be unblocked had to abandon hopes of becoming pregnant. Whilst surgery is now available, and its success has also increased in recent years, there is now the alternative of in-vitro fertilization (IVF) for those who cannot overcome this problem surgically.

IVF is a technique in which eggs are removed from the ovary, mixed with sperm in the laboratory and then, if fertilization occurs, are returned to the uterus two or three days later when the embryo is at the 4–8 cell stage.[24] Because more than one egg is required for this procedure the ovaries must be stimulated to produce a number of follicles. Eggs are collected from the folli-cles either by a laparoscopy – a surgeon can look into the pelvis with a small telescope during this procedure – or by direct removal of the contents of the follicles by a needle inserted through the wall of the abdomen, or via the vagina, with the help of an ultrasound scan to monitor the procedure. Eggs cannot be seen except under the microscope and thus are removed in the fluid inside each follicle. Eggs are graded for quality and placed in a culture medium in an incubator. Sperm, which has been washed, will be put in the culture containing the eggs and will be checked after about 18 hours to see if fertilization has occurred. Once the embryos (or more correctly pre-embryos) have divided into four or more cells they will be placed in the uterus via a fine tube inserted into the cervix.

Currently, in Britain, up to three fertilized eggs only are returned. In the past more embryos could be introduced and some authorities believe that, for the older women, limiting the number of returned embryos reduces the chances of a successful pregnancy. The limitation to three embryos was introduced to reduce the likelihood of multiple births but the latter (e.g. the risk of twins or triplets) has also been disputed as a risk for the older would-be mother in this context.[25] Once the fertilized egg is back in the uterus the rest of the development of the embryo parallels that of a naturally occurring pregnancy but some women may be given progesterone for a few weeks to support the pregnancy.

An IVF pregnancy can be identified by a blood test taken, typically, 14 days after embryo transfer. Success rates vary and individual clinics produce very different rates. One thing is certain; the older the woman the lower her chances of success. Women embarking on this form of treatment should expect to have several attempts – one attempt can be very costly and for women over 35 in Britain, the likelihood of treatment on the National Health is low. Planning for one treatment only, if funds are limited, places an enormous pressure on the woman and, if she fails to conceive, increases her desolation. Although a few women will conceive on their first attempt most will not and it is advisable to try to plan for several treatments if this procedure is to be attempted at all.

IVF is a treatment that is ideal for those who are ovulating but whose eggs cannot reach the uterus, but it can also be used to overcome the problems of a low sperm count since it saves the sperm the long journey to the egg. A variation on this treatment has been developed since the advent of IVF and this treatment is called gamete intrafallopian transfer or GIFT.

Gamete intrafallopian transfer

This procedure is suitable only for women who do not have blocked Fallopian tubes. It is a procedure rather like IVF, in that eggs are collected, but fertilization does not take place outside the woman's body.[24] Instead eggs (again, in Britain, not more than three) are placed with sperm into the Fallopian tube, and it is hoped fertilization will subsequently take place. Some authorities have now shown that the restriction to three eggs (or oocytes) in women over 40 undergoing GIFT reduces the chances of pregnancy in such women relative to that achieved prior to the restriction made by the Human Fertilization and Embryology Authority.[25] The risk of multiple pregnancy in this age group is low and it is suggested that the number restriction should be lifted for older women undergoing this procedure. GIFT may be appropriate for unexplained infertility in the woman and for males with a low sperm count. The success rate is said to be high – about a 21 per cent pregnancy rate but again it is lower in older women.[26,27]

Storing embryos

In both the above procedures spare eggs or embryos may result. In IVF any eggs in excess of three cannot be used and may be fertilized and frozen for use later. In GIFT spare eggs may be fertilized in the laboratory (just as in the IVF procedure) and also saved.

The possibility of storing eggs rather than embryos is now a real one and if a woman could store her own eggs when young this would overcome many of the problems of the older woman since her eggs would not have aged with her. A possible scenario could be that young women wishing to delay parenthood could store their eggs for use later – thereby avoiding the increased risks of genetic abnormalities well known for the 35-plus mother (*see Chapter 5*).

Other procedures

In addition to the two described here there are many other procedures – some of which are variations on these two forms of assisted conception. These will not all be discussed but suffice to say that these provide hope for a wide range of fertility problems.

Egg donation

If a woman does not produce her own eggs it is still possible for her to achieve a pregnancy with the use of donated eggs. The baby born will not be genetically hers but her body will have nurtured it throughout the pregnancy and it will, in this sense, feel just as much hers as would a 'normally achieved' pregnancy. The egg can be fertilized by her partner's sperm and thus the couple will have a baby that has one biological parent in the couple who raise it. In this sense it is exactly like the child of a couple who have had artifical insemination by donor, where the child is genetically related to one of its parents.

Egg donation, from the recipient's viewpoint, is quite a straightforward procedure. It is like the latter part of the IVF procedure where the fertilised egg, in the 4–8 cell stage, is inserted into the uterus via a tube through the cervix. The recipient may well require hormone treatment, firstly to ensure that the lining of the uterus is at its best, and later to support the pregnancy. For the donor of eggs the procedure is more complex – it is akin to the IVF procedure – because a woman's ovaries must be stimulated to produce a good crop of eggs and then these are collected as was described for IVF. Women volunteering eggs for use in this way have to undergo quite a lengthy treatment to produce the eggs. For this reason egg donors are rather more scarce than sperm donors. Sometimes eggs come from a woman undergoing sterilization who will donate eggs at the time of her sterilization operation; sometimes donors are relatives or friends of those who have experienced infertility and are aware of the devastation it can cause in the lives of those denied a baby. Some authorities believe that women should carry ovary donor cards to enable their eggs to be used in the event of their untimely death.[28]

In addition to the women who volunteer to donate eggs there is another potential source of eggs: the aborted foetus. Roger Gosden of Edinburgh University, Scotland, is interested in exploring this possibility.[29] He argues that if research could be carried out on such foetuses it might be possible to enable the foetus's eggs to be used to help the infertile. Currently, aborted embryos can be used for research in Britain for up to 14 days after conception, but there is a resistance in some quarters to the use of the 'eggs', or more correctly the 'fetal germ cells', of such embryos being the source of a new life.

There is a great need for egg donation amongst a number of groups of women: women with Turner's syndrome, a condition in which a woman lacks one X chromosome and, as a result, is unable to produce her own eggs; women who have an early menopause, and women who, as a result of conditions such as cancer or surgery, have had their ovaries removed. In addition to these women, some women who reach the menopause at the usual age of around 50 years may also wish for a baby, but egg donation for women past this stage has now become a controversial topic.

Much has been said about the rights and wrongs of egg donation at 50-plus, but it is undoubtedly a method of having a baby for some women who are otherwise fit and healthy. Michael Sauer in America and Severino Antinori in Italy have, as we pointed out in Chapter 2, helped a number of women over the age of 50 to achieve a pregnancy and all the indications are that the procedure is relatively simple.[30,31] An egg from a younger woman is fertilized and inserted into the uterus of the older woman who has been stimulated hormonally so that she can receive it. The young fertilized egg, now an embryo, has a good chance of successfully implanting itself in the wall of the uterus and developing normally. Most of the problems of the older mother prior to her menopause rest with her eggs, rather than the uterus and once hormones are used to stimulate the uterus, and a youthful egg has been provided, the outcome is often favourable.[27] The issue of whether women at 50-plus should be allowed this procedure is much debated. Mary Warnock, who chaired the Committee of Inquiry into Human Fertilization in 1982–84, believes, for instance, 'it is inherently wrong and offensive that a woman of 55 should have a child', and Robert Winston, Professor of Fertility Studies at the University of London Institute of Obstetrics and Gynaecology, has commented that 'the risks of pregnancy are very considerable in women over the age of fifty years'; but amongst those who have had the treatment clearly these problems do not necessarily arise.[32,33] As we have already seen in Chapter 2, approximately 50 women per year in

Britain over the age of 50 have a baby naturally. Are these women doing something *'inherently wrong and offensive'*? Furthermore, are these ageist attitudes responsible for the very high levels of terminations in women aged 40 and over (currently 42 per cent of all conceptions at this age), the highest figure for any age group of mothers, including mothers under the age of 20?[34]

A legal restriction on the basis of *age alone* seems to us, the authors, to be quite inappropriate. For both men and women we feel that other issues are more important than age in determining whether they 'should' or 'should not' become parents. Men father babies at any stage of life – Picasso was renowned for becoming a father twice over in his late sixties.[35] Reactions to later fatherhood are generally positive; often such men are thought to be especially virile and rarely if ever is there any discussion about the child's right to have a youthful father who will survive for the child's first two decades. The needs of the child are the same whether the mother or father is in middle or later life and, if we believe that a child has a right to have living parents most or all of his or her young life, then this should be applied equally to older men as to older women. If, on the other hand, we do not believe that we can legislate about such relationships, but merely encourage parents to be responsible, then the decision for the older mother should be left for her, her partner and the medical practitioner to whom the couple go for advice on later life parenthood. Ian Craft has commented:

> I absolutely believe cases must be decided individually and on their merits. If the Human Fertilization Embryology Authority brings in an upper age limit, it is going to deny somebody the chance of being helped, and that would be very sad.[36]

⤳

Miscarriage and age

Achieving conception does not guarantee a successful pregnancy; the risk of miscarriage, especially for the older woman, needs to be considered before hopes of a baby are raised too high.

Today any woman can buy an 'over the counter' pregnancy test that works virtually as soon as a period is missed; a 'clinical pregnancy' can be identified 14 days after ovulation. In past times women were often advised to wait for two missed periods (menses) before going to see their doctor about a possible pregnancy and thus such women were at, or after, 8 weeks gestation (or 6 weeks embryogenesis[37]) before they were recognized as pregnant. A slightly 'late' period would barely have been noticed yet it might have been a very early miscarriage.

Today, with the early identification of pregnancy the miscarriage rate appears to be on the increase, yet in part this is only due to the former lack of recognition of an early loss. This early recognition of pregnancy can be a mixed blessing because for those very eager to become pregnant it can cause much distress.

Rates of miscarriage by age vary from study to study. Research in the 1960s recorded rates of 12.2 per cent under the age of 20, 15.5 per cent at ages 30–34, 18.7 per cent at ages 35–39 and up to 25.5 per cent at age 40 and above.[38] In the 1980s John Hansen summarized the range of incidence by maternal age (*see Table 4.5*).[39] He noted that miscarriage rates increase by about 50 per cent from the twenties to the thirties and more rapidly to a two to four-fold increase for those above 40, compared with those in their twenties.

Table 4.5. Range of incidence of miscarriage by maternal age

Age in years	Range of incidence (%)
20–29	7.2–15
30–39	13.5–20.5
40 and over	21–46.1

Source: Hansen, 1986[38]

These figures are not a true reflection of the risk for an *individual* because there are several confounding factors. These include spontaneous abortion rate (i.e. some women are more likely to have miscarriages than others), the number of previous miscarriages (for each miscarriage the risk of another one increases slightly[40]), birth order and gravidity (for each birth, the miscarriage rate increases). Thus for each individual her particular gynaecological and obstetric history is crucial in determining for her the likelihood of a miscarriage in a current pregnancy.

Findings from women undergoing artificial insemination are again of relevance in this context. Such women are usually monitored from the time of treatment and hence the likely time of conception is accurately known unlike the situation for women who become pregnant naturally. Some Canadian research has reported on the outcome of 404 treatment courses in 330 couples.[41] A treatment course was defined as completed if the patient failed to conceive after 12 cycles, became pregnant (or dropped out). Twenty per cent dropped out and there were 42 spontaneous abortions amongst the 242 pregnancies (i.e. a 17 per cent miscarriage rate). The link with maternal age was clear – as can be seen in Table 4.6.

Table 4.6. Miscarriage rate in women undergoing artificial insemination

Age in years	Spontaneous abortions (%)
26–30	8
31–35	23
36 and older	30

Source: Virro & Shewchek, 1984[19]

Thus for women in their late thirties and older, miscarriage rates are raised. Again it should be noted that for all these studies the precise point at which a pregnancy is recognized will vary. Women receiving artificial insemination are likely to be tested for a pregnancy earlier than women in the population in general, thus early miscarriages – that might be mistaken for late periods in other groups – will be identified and hence inflate the figures.

To sum up, then; there is a risk of miscarriage in early pregnancy but to estimate a woman's likelihood of miscarriage requires a careful assessment of her own gynaecological and obstetric history. Women who have simply delayed trying for a baby until 35 or so and have no previous history of abortions (spontaneous or otherwise) are likely to have a *lower* risk of miscarriage than women who at age 35 have been trying to have a baby for some years and have a history of miscarriages.

~ 5 ~

What are the Risks? The Evidence on Problems associated with Later Motherhood

I wish that the fact that 97 per cent of children are born perfect had been stressed to me.

Woman in her forties looking back on her pregnancy

From the obstetrician's point of view a healthy woman of 38 is less of a risk than an unhealthy woman of 28.[1]

John Collee, Observer Magazine, 1991

The prospects for women having children after the age of 35 have never been better. Not only are women in this group generally more healthy than in the past, but improved medical technology has optimized the probability of a good outcome of pregnancy by providing interventions for those who do encounter difficulties and antenatal screening which gives information on the health of the expectant mother and her baby. Nevertheless, many women having a baby later are concerned whether they and particularly their baby will be 'all right'. This chapter looks at the evidence on the relationship between age and the health of mother and baby, including the risk of abnormalities such as Down's syndrome (*see Table 5.1*).[2,3,4,5,6] It reports on the screening and diagnostic procedures used to inform mothers of any such risks.

Table 5.1. Age of mother and risk of Down's syndrome (trisomy 21), Edward's syndrome (trisomy 18), Patau's syndrome (trisomy 13) and sex chromosome abnormalities (XXY or XXX) in the child

Mother's age	Risk at delivery of trisomy 21	Risk at amniocentesis of trisomy 21	trisomy 13 or 18	XXY or XXX
20	1/1923	–	–	–
25	1/1205	–	–	–
30	1/885	–	–	–
35	1/365	1/285	1/901	1/601
36	1/365	1/285	1/901	1/601
37	1/225	1/148	1/869	1/869
38	1/177	1/123	1/628	1/660
39	1/139	1/91	1/384	1/365
40	1/109	1/82	1/266	1/478
41	1/85	1/68	1/191	1/227
42	1/67	1/46	1/121	1/158
43	1/53	1/31	1/119	1/159
44	1/41	1/34	1/203	1/112
45	1/32	1/22	1/169	1/7

Sources: 1. Donnal, D. (1988). 'Genetic Risk' in D. K. James & G.M. Stirratt (Eds) *Pregnancy and Risk*, John Wiley & Sons.
2. James, D.K. (1988). 'Risk at booking' in D.K. James & G.M. Stirratt (Eds) *Pregnancy and Risk*, John Wiley & Sons.

༅

Studies of medical risk: some important questions

The number of studies which have been conducted to assess the obstetric and neonatal risk associated with the age of the mother exceeds 100. These studies have taken place over many years (1917–94) and the range of methods they have used has varied greatly. Because the age of a study and the methods it uses affect its quality, and therefore the value that can be placed on its findings, it is important to begin by taking a closer look at the way each study was done. There are a number of key questions:

How old is the study?

Because there have been historical changes in the reasons why women have babies later (*see Chapter 2*) the age of a study is an important consideration. In the past the group of women who had babies after 35 was made up primarily of women with larger families who were continuing to have children beyond the age of 35, and those who had experienced fertility problems. Today a very different group of women is having children after the age of 35. Later mothers are now more likely to be women who have voluntarily delayed first-time parenthood or who are completing smaller families. Large numbers of pregnancies and fertility problems are risk factors in their own right. Because of this, older studies of motherhood after 35, particularly those done prior to 1970, are of a different and more 'at-risk' population than those which are more recent.

The reasons for women having babies later is not the only historical change. Medical technology and obstetric practice are constantly developing. Screening has enabled the more accurate targeting of services to the women who require special antenatal care and there have been wide ranging developments in obstetrical knowledge and practice. This means that some factors which were once associated with adverse outcome of pregnancy are no longer associated in this way. Older studies will not reflect these developments. For a woman interested in the risk of having a baby after 35 in the 1990s more recent studies are obviously likely to be most relevant, and those involving the largest number of participants will give the most accurate picture.

How many women were studied?

If we are to be able to generalize from the findings of a study there should be a large number of women studied and they should be representative of the type of women that normally have children after 35.

There are two main reasons why larger numbers make for a better study. Firstly, the type of outcomes that these studies are interested in such as maternal death, complications of pregnancy, neonatal death and congenital abnormality are relatively rare. If they are found to happen in a small group this could just be a chance finding and may lead to an inflated estimate of the risk to older mothers. More commonly, no incidence of this outcome will be found and the risk cannot be assessed. Only large studies are able to look at rarer outcomes with any degree of accuracy. Secondly, a wide diversity of women now have babies after 35 and to represent this broad range a large number would need to be studied. In general the larger the number of women studied the greater is the value of the study.

What sort of women were studied?

Demographic studies suggest that certain groups are more likely to have a later pregnancy; thus there are likely to be some biases in a representative sample of today's later mothers – there would be more professional women, for example. Because the reasons for women having children later vary it is also important to look at the different medical risk for sub-groups. Most importantly studies should consider the role of four key variables:

parity (the number of children a woman has had) – because first-time mothers and women who have had a large number of children are at an increased risk regardless of age.[2,5]

obstetric history (whether a woman has experienced fertility problems, miscarriages or termination of pregnancy) – those who have had miscarriages, fertility problems or have had more pregnancies are at higher risk regardless of age.[2,5]

medical history and pre-existing medical conditions – some diseases increase the risk of problems during pregnancy and, though not directly a result of age, are more advanced with age.[2]

multiple birth – twinning increases with age and is a high risk factor but is not directly a result of age.[7,8]

In assessing whether the findings of a particular study are relevant to any one woman it is important for that woman to consider how similar her demographic (e.g. race, class, age) and obstetric (e.g. first-time pregnancy versus second or more) characteristics are to those of the women studied. The more similar they are the greater the likelihood that the findings have personal relevance.

What is the study actually looking at?

There are many factors which may affect pregnancy outcome which change with age but which are not actually caused by age. These are called covariates. For example, a woman who is a smoker will have a longer history of smoking if she is older and although smoking is not caused by her being older, her longer history of smoking may be an increased risk to her pregnancy. Similarly some medical conditions are not a result of being older but are exacerbated by it (e.g. hypertension and diabetes). Studies which have a sufficiently large number of women to study and which collect information on these covariates are able to distinguish how any risk to the mother or her baby is due to her age or to the factors which change with age. This is important because while age is something that cannot be changed, intervention (e.g. stopping smoking, or education) can reduce the risk associated with the covarying risk factor. *Studies which do not distinguish age from its covariates may not be studying the risk of age at all but rather the effects of other factors.*

What do the findings mean?

The results of studies examining the risk of increasing age on the mother and child are typically reported as a *relative risk*. They compare the rates of a range of adverse outcomes for the mother (pre-eclampsia, gestational diabetes, prolonged labour, assisted delivery, Caesarean section, maternal mortality) and child (congenital abnormality, pre-term birth, low birthweight, still-birth, neonatal death) with those of other groups. If the rates of these adverse outcomes are higher then the relative risk will be higher. In some studies this is expressed as a percentage increase in risk relative to a comparison group. The comparison groups vary. In some studies comparisons are made with a range of different age bands but in others the comparison is made with just one other age band. This is typically the age 20–25 which is thought to be physiologically the optimal age for reproduction. The effect of this is to give a higher relative risk figure. Comparison with age bands 26–30 and 31–35 will therefore give lower risk figures.

It is also important to recognize the distinction between *relative* and *absolute* risk. While studies may report an inflated or high risk of adverse outcome, the actual (absolute) risk may be low. A good example here is that of the risk of Down's syndrome (trisomy 21). Table 5.1 presents the risk for this condition by age. The risk increases considerably by age from one in 1900 at 20 years to one in 32 at 45 years. At 35 the risk is one in 365. The relative risk is high – four times higher than that for a 20 year-old – but the actual risk is still low – more than 99 per cent of babies will not have Down's syndrome. To put this in context: a guideline used following screening tests is that conclusive prenatal diagnosis using invasive procedures such as amniocentesis need not be recommended unless the risk is one in 200.[2] A woman's risk at 35 is about half this. Thus it is important to realize that a raised risk relative to other groups does not necessarily mean a high risk in absolute terms. Chapter 6 discusses women's own experiences of dealing with decisions about these concepts, and describes alternative ways of expressing information about relative and absolute risk.

In summary, when considering the medical research on the risks of problems associated with pregnancy and birth beyond the age of 35 it is important to take account of the quality of the study, which is affected by its age, the size of the group of women studied, the characteristics of the women studied, whether it analyses for sub-groups and whether it accounts for covariates. *The risk to the health of mother and baby may be high relative to other groups but still very low in absolute terms.*

⬦

What are the risks to the mother's health?

Risks in pregnancy and childbirth

Studies examining the effect of age on a mother's health during pregnancy and at the birth have considered a range of health outcomes. Principal among these are pregnancy loss (miscarriage), pregnancy-induced hypertension (toxaemia), placental complications, prolonged labour, delivery by Caesarean section and maternal death.

MISCARRIAGE

Miscarriage is a loss of the foetus prior to 24 weeks of gestation. It is estimated that up to a third of pregnancies result in a miscarriage though many of these are undetected because the woman is unaware that she is pregnant (*see Chapter 4*). Most miscarriages occur in the first trimester of pregnancy.

Research has consistently reported that with increasing maternal age there are higher rates of miscarriage (*see Table 4.5 –* Chapter 4).[9,10] It is possible that this is a failure of implantation but in view of the findings of higher levels of chromosomal errors occurring at ovulation in the older woman (*see Box 5.1*) it is likely that a greater proportion of these are accounted for by early foetal death resulting from abnormality rather than gynaecological or physiological problems.[4]

HYPERTENSION/PRE-ECLAMPSIA

Eclampsia is a life-threatening condition for both mother and baby which typically occurs late in pregnancy. Its name derives from the Greek and means 'like a flash of lightning' because it is characterized by the experience of flashing lights, fits and eventually coma. It is life-threatening to the foetus because the uterus goes into spasm and restricts blood flow, and to the mother because it causes kidney failure, lowering of oxygen to the brain and haemorrhages to tissue such as the liver. This condition is now rare in the Western world but its precondition, pre-eclampsia, is not. Pre-eclampsia is estimated to occur in about 15 per cent of all pregnancies.[11] Pre-eclampsia is characterized by the swelling of the face, hands and feet (oedema), elevated blood pressure and protein in the urine. It most frequently occurs in first-time pregnancies.

A number of studies have reported higher rates of pre-eclampsia in older expectant women compared with younger controls. Some of these reports are for women over 35,[12-15] while others are for women over 40.[16-19] There has also been one study which reports increased risk for women who have already had children previously but not for first-time mothers[22] and one in which no differences were found.[23] The quality of studies and the reporting of increased hypertension/pre-eclampsia vary and cannot be considered conclusive but they do suggest some increased risk with age. The type of women studied has varied also. Notably, the two studies which found no increased risk for first-time mothers were of a white, middle-class, highly educated group of women over 35.

PLACENTAL COMPLICATIONS

There are three major groups of placental complications which are typically considered:

> *placental separation* (*abruptio placentae*) – the placenta partially or completely separates from the uterus causing vaginal bleeding

in about a half to one per cent of pregnancies. The cause of this is unknown but it occurs more commonly in women who have had two or more children.

placenta praevia – this occurs when the placenta is embedded in the lower segment of the uterus rather than the upper segment. It is a major cause of vaginal bleeding after the twentieth week of pregnancy and of haemorrhage in the final two months. The cause is unknown but it is more common in women who have had several children.

placental insufficiency – because the placenta is the developing baby's source of oxygen and nourishment the health of the placenta is critical. Placental insufficiency may be signalled by poor growth of the foetus, low rate of activity of the foetus and low fundal height which indicates that the uterus is not expanding at the expected rate.

General obstetric texts report that both placental separation and placenta praevia may increase with maternal age but evidence from studies which specifically examine complications of pregnancy in women over 35 is less conclusive.[2] One study of a predominantly white, middle-class group of women over 35 which was conducted between 1981 and 1983 did not find a raised risk for either in first or subsequent pregnancies.[20] Another of a middle-class but racially mixed group over the age of 35 conducted from 1985–87 reports that there were more pregnancy complications compared with younger women. Placental complications were among the potential problems considered by this study but these alone were not significantly raised.[21] The most recent study, conducted between 1988 and 1991, which was of a white, predominantly middle-class population found no differences in placental problems between mothers over 35 and those in the age groups 20–29 or 30–34.[22] Only one study reports a significantly increased risk of placental complications.[18] This study, conducted in 1977, was of a very different group of women; they were over the age of 40, predominantly black and of low socio-economic status and high parity (72 per cent had more than four children and 18 per cent of these had more than 13 children).

It may be that the reports in general texts are based on older studies and are picking up the effect of parity. Women with more than two children are more likely to experience placental complications and, of course, women with more children will be older. In more recent studies the group of older expectant mothers studied are typically having their first or second child and a finding of placental complications is less likely. The evidence from the most recently conducted studies which are of middle-class women having their first child or a subsequent child in a small family over 35 is that risk of placental complication is not significantly increased for this group.

PROLONGED LABOUR

A labour is said to be prolonged if progress toward delivery of the baby is slow and contractions fail to bring about delivery. There are two main reasons why this occurs. Firstly, the cervix may dilate slowly if the uterus does not contract efficiently. Secondly, there may be an obstruction which prevents the baby descending. Obstruction may occur because of the position of the baby or because of the size of the baby relative to that of the mother. Prolonged labour can result in maternal exhaustion and cause distress to the foetus. Often it results in higher levels of analgesia and assisted delivery – forceps and ventouse extraction and Caesarean section. It is more common in first-time deliveries.[11]

The notion that older women are more likely to have prolonged labours presumably derives from the theory that an older body and, particularly an older uterus, is less efficient. A number of studies report an increased duration of labour in older mothers,[21-26] but at least as many report no such increase.[19,27-30] One study reports reduced duration of labour with age.[33] This study cannot be taken as reliable, however, since it did not control for parity (first versus subsequent deliveries). The finding reflects the well-documented reduction in duration of labour in subsequent deliveries rather than the effect of age.

Two of the studies finding an association of increased duration of labour with age are quite dated and methodologically limited.

One of these studied only women over the age of 40 and the other women over the age of 44. The other three, however, warrant further consideration. Ian Morrison looked at the medical records of 127 women having their first baby over the age of 35. He reports that the average length of labour was 11 hours for those who were not induced but that the length of labour was longer for the group in general. Some 38 per cent of his study group were induced.[25] Wayne Cohen and colleagues, in examining the length of labour in older mothers, considered the effects of use of pain relief, particularly epidural anaesthesia. This study reports an increase in prolonged labour in first-time mothers over the age of 35 even when pain relief was taken into account. The comparison group for this study, however, was of women under the age of 20. No differences with women in other age groups were reported.[26] The recent study of first time mothers over the age of 35 by Gertrud Berkowitz and colleagues focused on the duration of the second stage of labour which is the period between full dilation of the cervix and delivery of the baby. She found that women having their first child over 35 were more likely to have a long second stage (greater than two hours) even when they took account of race and the use of epidural anaesthesia.[21] The age and range of studies which have found no differences between length of labour of older and younger mothers vary but they do include recent studies which have satisfactory methodologies and representative samples.

Currently the evidence concerning the relationship between maternal age and duration of labour is not conclusive. The use of anaesthesia can increase the duration of labour, however, and higher rates of anaesthetic intervention have been found in the older age group.[20] Similarly, induction of labour will increase duration of labour and the rates of intervention are higher for older women.[25,20] The reason for this intervention is unclear but it is possible that some explanation for this is not so much the mother's physical capabilities to deal with labour but concern on the part of both mother and obstetrician about the older, 'at risk', status of bearing a child after 35.

CAESAREAN SECTION

The rates of Caesarean section delivery have been consistently found to be higher among women having a child over the age of 35 than among younger women.[13,14,19,20,22] The studies reporting these increased rates include the two most recent studies which have sound methods and their findings are likely to be reliable.

The reasons for this increase in Caesarean section rate are complex. Caesarean section usually follows complications at delivery, but the rates of Caesarean in women over 35 exceed the rate we would expect given the figure on complications of delivery. The recent study of Jeffery Peipert and Michael Bracken found that women over the age of 35 with no complications of pregnancy or labour were twice as likely to have their child delivered by Caesarean section than women in younger age groups.[22] Again it is likely that this finding reflects the greater caution of both the obstetrician and the mother. However, analysis of the hospital records of the 107 participants in the Leicester Motherhood Project revealed that rates of Caesarean section were not higher in this study for the women over 35 than they were for the comparison group of women in their twenties.[32] This very recent prospective study recruited every 35-plus first-time mother-to-be at a Leicester antenatal clinic who was willing to take part over a certain period (half of those initially approached) and selected comparison groups so that levels of education and occupational status were the same in both age groups. Because of the characteristics of the target group of 35-plus first-time mothers, these findings may be particularly relevant for highly-educated women with non-manual occupations.

Obstetricians unaware of recent studies to the contrary may believe that women over the age of 35 are at high risk and therefore be more inclined to opt for a Caesarean delivery. The woman herself may also be concerned about her 'risk status' and more inclined to accept a premature decision to deliver by Caesarean.[22,33]

MATERNAL DEATH

Maternal death is now, thankfully, a very rare event indeed. Because the number of maternal deaths is small it is difficult to study the role maternal age plays. The Report of the Confidential Enquiry into Maternal Deaths in the United Kingdom for 1988 – 90 indicates that among women who die as a result of child-bearing there is a higher proportion of women over the age of 35, and particularly over the age of 40.[35] Other studies which have been conducted over the past 30 years which have considered maternal death as well as other factors do not provide conclusive evidence for an association with later motherhood.[12,14,34]

Long term risks to health

In addition to health immediately associated with pregnancy and childbirth some studies have examined long-term risks associated with later motherhood, in particular the risk of breast and uterine cancer.

BREAST CANCER

Findings concerning the risk of breast cancer suggest that child-bearing is 'better late than never'. A higher incidence of breast cancer is reported for women who have not borne children than for those who have.[36,37] Among women who do have children, the age of child-bearing may be an important factor.

More than 40 years ago it was noted that married women over the age of 35 who had children had a lower rate of death due to breast cancer than both married and unmarried woman of the same age who did not have children. However, below the age of 35 it was found that women who had children were at higher risk.[38] It was suggested that the explanation for this was that pregnancy had two effects on breast tissue. In the short-term pregnancy has a deleterious effect which makes it more suscep-tible to cancer but in the long term it has a protective effect. The short-term increased risk is likely to be a result of increased estro-gens in pregnancy.[39] Several studies have subsequently examined the association between breast cancer, pregnancy and women's age.

Following the findings of the early studies[38] some have exam-ined the risk of breast cancer in relation to the *interval* between age of the mother and her age at last full-term pregnancy[44] but others have examined the relationship between the *actual age* of the mother at first or last full-term pregnancy instead.[45,46] Studies looking at the interval between age at last pregnancy and breast cancer have been inconclusive. While some report that risk of breast cancer increases in the short-term others have found no association.[40] Studies of the effect of maternal age itself are simi-larly inconclusive. A large multi-centre study conducted since the 1960s has suggested that the age at first pregnancy is important with women having children after the age of 30 being at increased risk of breast cancer.[45] The mechanisms for this are unknown, however, and the relationship with other factors such as the number of children the woman bears unclear. A recent study suggests that it is age at last pregnancy which is the important predictor of breast cancer and also that having a larger family protects against breast cancer. This study argues that it is the reduction in family size which explains the observed increase in the rates of breast cancer in the general population and not the trends to delayed childbearing.[40]

The findings on the relationship between age at first and last birth and breast cancer are difficult to interpret. The effect is likely to be transitory, however. It has been found that after the meno-pause any protective effect of having had children diminishes.[47]

UTERINE CANCER

In terms of uterine cancer later motherhood is beneficial. Studies of endometrial uterine cancer have consistently found that women having children later are at *decreased* risk of this disease.[48,49] Gunnar Kvale and colleagues suggest this is because a pregnancy results in a mechanical exfoliation of the uterus at delivery which will remove any cells in early or late stage of malignant transformation.[50]

ح⁓

What are the risks for the child?

Risk to the foetus and young baby

Studies which look at the effect of the mother's age use a range of outcomes to gauge its impact on the health of the child from the antenatal period through to the early weeks of life. Primary among these are: pre-term birth, birthweight, health at delivery, perinatal and neonatal death, and congenital abnormality.

PRE-TERM DELIVERY

A pre-term delivery is one which occurs before 37 completed weeks of gestation. Pre-term birth presents a threat to the health of the infant, though typically it is the very pre-term infant born before 33 weeks gestation who is at the greatest risk of long-term poor health. Studies examining pre-term delivery as an outcome tend only to report on whether or not the child was born prior to 37 weeks gestation so this is only a crude measure of the child's health. Additionally, it should be noted that to know whether a child is pre-term depends upon accurately dating the conception of the child and a range of variables will affect the accuracy of this. A woman who conceives as a result of fertility treatment, for example, will have precise dates while an unplanned conception to a woman with an irregular menstrual cycle will be less accurately dated.

In studies which do not take account of factors which covary with age and which affect the occurrence of pre-term delivery, particularly obstetric history, smoking and pre-pregnancy health of mother, increased rates of pre-term birth are reported for women over the age of 35.[15,51-53] Recent studies which have been more careful to take account of these factors do not find differences in the rate of pre-term birth.[14,19-22] Susan Barken and Michael Bracken[56] in a study of more than 1300 first time mothers found that the rates of pre-term birth were higher but when other important factors were taken into account this was not a significant difference.[54] The methodologically sound study of Gertrud Berkowitz and colleagues found no increase in the rate of pre-term delivery in their study of almost 4000 first-time mothers and for women over the age of 40 they found a slightly lower rate of pre-term birth.[21] The weight of recent evidence suggests that age does not constitute an increased risk for pre-term birth.

ABNORMAL BIRTHWEIGHT

A baby's birthweight is often used as a measure of the health of the baby at birth. Low birthweight is generally defined as below 2500 grams and babies who are of low birthweight typically are not as healthy. Low birthweight occurs if a baby is born pre-term or has failed to develop well in the uterus (small for gestational age). High birthweight (macrosomy) has also been considered in some studies. High birthweight is a sign of gestational diabetes and may result in problems at delivery but is not usually a threat to the health of the baby in its own right.

Most recent studies of the birthweight of babies born to women over 35 compared with younger mothers do not provide evidence for a risk of low birthweight. For first-time mothers many studies report no differences when compared with younger age groups.[14,20,54] Gertrud Berkowitz and colleagues, however, found more low birthweight babies were born to women over the age of 35.[23] Two studies report a higher rate of exceptionally big (macrosomic) babies occurring in women having a subsequent baby over the age of 35.[19,20]

POOR HEALTH AT DELIVERY

At one minute and five minutes after the birth of a baby a series of observations are made on the baby to assess his or her health. The observations include pulse rate, breathing pattern, movements, skin colour, and reflexes. On the basis of these a score, called an Apgar score, is given to convey a general picture of the baby's health. The maximum score is 10 and most babies score between 7 and 10. To assess the impact of mother's age on the health of the baby at birth three studies have looked at Apgar scores. Ian Morrison and Gertrud Berkowitz both considered the number of babies born with Apgar scores lower than 7 to women having their first child but their findings conflict.[25,21] In the Morrison study women over 35 had a higher number with low Apgar scores while in the Berkowitz study they had slightly fewer. The explanation of these conflicting findings is probably associated with the timing of the studies and the methods they used. The Berkowitz study is considerably more recent (18 years) and is of a much larger group of women (3917 versus 127) and is therefore more likely to be reliable. Donna Kirz reports that women expecting subsequent children over the age of 35 had a higher number of babies receiving an Apgar score less than 4 but, in support of the findings of Gertrud Berkowtiz, that this was not evident among first-born babies to women over 35.[20]

Rates of admission to neonatal intensive care has also been used by these studies as a measure to assess the health of the baby. Again there are conflicting findings. While Donna Kirz and colleagues found fewer such admissions, both Gertrud Berkowtiz and Ian Morrison report higher rates of admission.

One small study which has looked at the behaviour of new-born infants has suggested babies of older mothers are less healthy.[55]

INFANT DEATH

Rates of death prior to the birth (stillbirth), after the onset of labour (perinatal death) and in the first week of life (neonatal death) have been considered in relation to maternal age by seven studies. Three studies, notably those which account for the effects of covariates, report no differences in the rates of still-birth, perinatal or neonatal death. Three studies report increases in stillbirth.[19,52,53] Michele Forman and colleagues found higher rates of stillbirth in women over the age of 35 compared with women in the age group 20–25.[52] Of these deaths 85 per cent were late foetal deaths occurring prior to delivery. John Keily and colleagues, in a comparison with women aged 20–29, report a similar finding and attribute this to higher rates of foetal abnor-mality.[53] William Spellacy and colleagues studied births to women over 40 only.[19] In this group they found higher rates of foetal death but these were reported to be a result of existing hypertension and high multiparity (having many previous chil-dren) than the age of the mother as such. Leon Israel and J. Deutschberger's now quite dated study found higher rates of death around the time of delivery but this was only among the group of women having a first child over the age of 40.[31] Since this study had few controls there may be many factors not related to age that explain the findings.

It would seem that risk of perinatal or neonatal death are not appreciably raised for children born to mothers over the age of 35. The evidence on foetal death prior to the onset of labour is less conclusive but may be higher if the mother has medical prob-lems such as hypertension or if the infant has an abnormality.

ABNORMALITY

Chromosomal abnormality resulting from failure of separation of a chromosome pair from one of the parents (trisomies) are the most commonly reported abnormality related to later mother-hood (*see Box 5.1*). Of these Down's syndrome (trisomy 21) is the most commonly known but there is also evidence for increased incidence of Edward's syndrome (trisomy 18) and Patau syndrome (trisomy 13).[2,3,6] These all result in intellectual impair-ment of the child. Abnormalities arising from non-disjunction of the sex chromosome, particularly Klinefelter syndrome (XXY) and Triple X syndrome (XXX), have also been found to increase with advanced maternal age.[3,6] Such abnormalities are associated with sterility and may have associated behavioural abnormality. The findings of the relationship between these abnormalities and maternal age is consistently reported and accepted as reliable. The risk of their occurrence gradually increases with age. The risk of Down's syndrome is the greatest and this drops to below one in 200 at the age of 38. At this age diagnostic screening, using amniocentesis or chorionic villus sampling, has been advocated for obstetric practice.[2]

One major recent study of the association between later motherhood and non-chromosomal birth defects has found that older mothers are at lower risk. Patricia Baird and colleagues studied over half a million births in British Colombia between 1966 and 1981.[56] Among this group of children, once chromosomal abnormalities were excluded, 43 different types of birth defect occurred. The authors looked to see if the rate of any of these 43 abnormalities were associated with the age of the child's mother. They found associations of mothers' age with three types of defect: patent ductus arteriosus, hypertrophic pyloric stenosis and congenital dislocatable hip. Contrary to what might be popularly expected, in all three conditions the rate for children born to mothers over the age of 35 was lower than for younger maternal age groups.

Long-term health outcomes

There have been sporadic reports of associations between maternal age and longer-term health outcomes. Both schizophrenia and leukaemia have been linked to maternal age, though the reasons for this are unknown.[57,58] Higher rates of both anorexia and school phobia have also been reported among children of older mothers but again the reasons for this are unknown.[59]

WHY MIGHT THERE BE AN INCREASED RISK OF ABNORMALITY? (BOX 5.1)

Most women know that there is an increased risk of chromosomal abnormality in babies born to older mothers (*Table 5.1*). Why should this be?

Well before a female human baby is born her total store of potential eggs are in place. These potential eggs are stored at a stage in which there are pairs of chromosomes until ovulation occurs in the adult female. Before ovulation, because the chromosomes will join with those of the male, separation of the chromosome pair occurs so that only a single chromosomal string should be contained in the released ovum.[4,5] Occasionally errors occur in this process leading to an abnormality in the developing baby. There are two types of error. Firstly, there may be a failure of the chromosomes to pair, resulting in a monosomy – a missing chromosome. Abnormalities occurring from monosomies usually cause the developing baby to die and will result in a miscarriage or stillbirth. Secondly, the chromosome pair from the ovum may fail to separate resulting in a trisomy or extra chromosome. Abnormalities occurring from trisomies less frequently cause death of the developing baby. Babies born with trisomies typically have intellectual impairment and abnormalities of physical appearance. The most commonly occurring and most commonly known trisomic condition is Down's syndrome (trisomy 21). However there are others such as Edward's syndrome (trisomy 18) and Patau's syndrome (trisomy 13) as well as those associated with the sex hormones, Klinefelter's syndrome (XXY) and Triple X syndrome (XXX).

Errors in the separation of chromosomes can occur in a woman at any age in her reproductive life. Why do they occur more frequently in older women?

The precise reason for the increase in chromosomal abnormalities with the age of the mother is not known but there are a number of possible reasons. One commonly suggested reason is that potential eggs are not all perfect at birth and that those that are defective are ovulated later in life – 'best eggs go first'. Another suggestion is that the egg store of an older woman has been subjected to a longer period of adverse environmental exposures which damage a once perfect potential egg. Yet another suggests that hormonal changes which occur later in a woman's reproductive life influence the process of ovulation, causing delayed ovulation and resulting in 'over-ripeness'. It may also be that defects in the potential egg, whatever the cause, are combined with reduced ability of the

cont.

uterus to select out defective embryos.[5] Currently, the greatest amount of evidence supports a hormonal cause. The explanation is unlikely to be simple but rather due to an interaction of a number of these factors.

Overview: is later motherhood 'risky'?

In 1988 Mansfield conducted an extensive review of the studies of the medical risk associated with later motherhood.[60] She concluded that the majority (61 per cent) of the studies were methodologically inadequate and that their conclusions which indicated increased risk for older mothers were of questionable value. Our own review has re-examined many of the studies reviewed by Mansfield but also the most recent studies in the period 1988–94. These more recent studies are generally well conducted: they examine large data sets containing information on a large number of women and their babies; they use more sophisticated methods of analysis which allow them to tease out the effects of maternal age from other factors which vary with age and, most importantly, they are of today's older mothers, in the western world, who are typically well-nourished, healthy and of low parity (have small numbers of children). What do we conclude?

The general picture is encouraging for the so-called 'elderly' mother (*see Box 5.2*). For healthy women who do not live in adverse circumstances and who are having a first child or completing a small family there are few increased risks to their own health compared with women under the age of 35. There is a likelihood of greater medical intervention – induction of labour, use of pain relief and Caesarean section – but these possibly reflect caution resulting from a belief on the part of both medical staff and the woman herself that later motherhood is risky, as much as an actual risk of being older. For the child the risk of having a chromosomal abnormality, particularly Down's syndrome (trisomy 21) is increased and this is particularly so after

---

WHAT'S IN A NAME?
'ELDERLY PRIMIPARAE', 'ELDERLY MULTIPARAE'
(BOX 5.2)

Because having children later is commonly believed to be a 'risk' to the health of mother and baby, the terms 'elderly primiparae' (for first-time mothers) and 'elderly multiparae' (for women who are already mothers) are used by medical staff to designate this special status. For a woman having a child after 35 it may seem strange or even offensive to be termed 'elderly'. Certainly, the term carries a negative under-tone suggesting not only risk but of failing to be 'on-time'.

Interestingly, the age at which a woman is termed 'elderly' by health professionals has changed in recent times. Ten years ago a woman of 30 having her first child would be termed elderly. Publi-cations such as *Birth Over Thirty* by Sheila Kitzinger singled out 30 as an age above which a woman holds a different status.[67] In more recent times 35 has become the age at which a woman is designated as elderly if she is expecting a child. Given that risk is not so much a function of age but rather relates to individual health and medical background the usefulness of such terms should be questioned.

---

a maternal age of 38; this risk, though increased, is still small in absolute terms below the age of 40. The findings on the relation-ship between later motherhood and other aspects of the child's health are less conclusive but again are likely to relate to the health and circumstance of the mother.

The picture for each individual woman will vary with her personal history. Screening and diagnostic testing, however can provide more information.

༄

Screening and diagnostic tests

Routine checks to monitor the mother's health

During pregnancy a number of routine screening procedures are undertaken to enable early detection of health problems for the mother. Regular checks of blood pressure and urine are made so that any conditions such as hypertension and diabetes can be detected and medical intervention be undertaken to minimize their impact.

Tests for abnormality in the baby

Screens are also available to detect foetal abnormality. These include routine ultrasound and screening of blood samples. Routine ultrasound is conducted between 16 and 18 weeks of a pregnancy. The scan will give a picture of the physical structure of the foetus and give an indication of abnormality particularly of the head or spine. Though it is not necessarily routine, blood tests to detect risk of abnormality are available. Most common of these is the alpha-fetoprotein (AFP) test which is performed at about 16 to 18 weeks of pregnancy. This test examines the level of alpha-fetoprotein, a protein from the baby, in the mother's blood. If the level of this protein is higher than normal there is an increased risk of spina bifida and if it is lower than normal an increased chance of Down's syndrome. Usually this test is combined with ultrasound results to give more definite information on the foetus. More recently the AFP test has been combined with tests for other chemicals in the blood to give a personal risk figure for Down's syndrome. This combined test is variously called the triple test or Bart's test. The risk figure presented will also take account of the mother's age.[61]

If a woman is thought to be at high risk of having a baby with an abnormality, particularly chromosomal abnormalities, spina bifida or genetically transmitted disorders, then more accurate diagnostic testing using amniocentesis can be conducted. This involves inserting a long needle into the uterus via the abdomen (with ultrasound for guidance) so that a small amount of amniotic fluid can be withdrawn. This fluid contains foetal cells which are then grown in a culture so that chromosomal and inborn metabolic disorders can be detected. This test is typically offered if a woman is over the age of 35 (in some hospitals) or 38 (in others), has a family history of the relevant abnormalities or has an ultrasound, AFP or triple test result which suggests there is a high risk. The results on spina bifida are available in a few days but for chromosomal abnormalities the results take up to four weeks.

An alternative test to detect chromosomal and genetic abnormalities, but not spina bifida, is chorionic villus sampling (CVS). This is carried out at 8 to 12 weeks of pregnancy. It involves aspiration of a small amount of chorionic villi, the tissue developing around the placenta, from which chromosomal analysis can be performed. The results of this test are available in a few days. Both amniocentesis and CVS present a risk of miscarriage. For amniocentesis this is about 0.5 per cent and for CVS this is 2 to 3 per cent.[2] In Chapter 1 we reported a case of CVS subsequently causing miscarriage. Chapter 6 contains further information on women's subjective experiences of these tests and the decision-making surrounding them.

The screening technology available is becoming increasingly more sophisticated and can reveal some abnormalities early enough for women to decide whether to continue with their pregnancies. However, they present the older woman with a new set of difficult choices and may present problems in their own right. A woman considering amniocentesis is faced with the choice between identification of abnormality and the potential miscarriage of a healthy baby. There is also a possibility, though small, of a false diagnosis and termination of a normal foetus. The woman is faced with ethical issues concerning the value of an abnormal foetus and the role of abortion. The ethical issues and the actual procedures may cause stress for an older woman and may affect her relationship with her baby in the early stage of pregnancy before test results are known.[62,32] On the other hand, the tests raise expectations that if no genetic abnormality is found the baby will be perfect.[63-66]

Advice on these decisions tends to come from the medical perspective which places an overriding emphasis on the achievement of a problem-free pregnancy and birth and a perfect baby. Prior to a decision to have a baby after 35 advice is typically pessimistic with warnings of the risk of later motherhood. After conception there is a pressure to accept the screening available to ensure a perfect baby. There are, however, women who do not

wish to reject an 'imperfect' baby. As advances in prenatal diagnosis have occurred there has been greater pressure on women
who do not choose to use them or who do not wish to act on the
information they provide.[59]

The experience for a woman having a baby after the age of 35
may not match the expectation of the medical perspective.
Women's own accounts are examined in the next chapter.

6

Pregnancy after 35: The Experience

I'm really pleased but I still can't believe it. I did a test at home but I didn't believe it till I got one done at the chemist's ... and then I was so dazed I forgot to pay.

Beryl, 38, first pregnancy

I was devastated. I thought it was the menopause at first. I did think about abortion: all my friends thought I was mad, my parents are old-fashioned, I didn't want to get rid of my horse. But it's not its [the baby's] fault, and now I've found a way to keep the horse I thought 'sod 'em all, I'll do what I want'.

Marie, 38, unplanned first pregnancy

What is it like to go through pregnancy after 35? Are older women more tired? Do they meet with different reactions because of their age, when they announce their pregnancies? What about antenatal screening – do older women worry more, or less, about themselves and their babies? Does age make any difference to how easy it is to adjust to pregnancy and to the idea of becoming a mother? These and many other questions will be explored during this chapter.

ﾂ

Reactions to becoming pregnant

How do women of 35-plus feel when they discover they are pregnant? One strand of thought is that the majority of babies conceived at this age may be carefully planned and therefore wanted. However, as at any age, this is not true for every mother as we pointed out in Chapter 3. For instance, the British study of 40-plus mothers found that in those taking part less than half the babies born to women over 40 were 'planned'.[1] Studies described in Chapter 3 suggest that women in their thirties may more often have planned pregnancies than women in their forties.

Feelings about pregnancy depend more on each woman's individual circumstances than just upon her age. However, for women who become pregnant accidentally, awareness that 'the biological clock is ticking away' may bring a new element into consideration: the pregnancy may be seen as a last chance to have another baby. As Maureen, introduced in Chapter 1, said at mid-pregnancy:

> *Once my marriage was over I felt as though I'd got nothing. I've got plenty of material things but they didn't mean anything to me. At first when I got pregnant I thought 'What've I done? How will I cope?' Now I just think it's fine . . . it was meant to be . . . after my mother died last year it was as if everything I loved had been taken away from me. Pregnancy has given me something to carry on for.*
>
> *Age 41, unplanned first baby*

In the British study of 40-plus mothers, although many of the babies were not planned, over two-thirds of the women were happy about the discovery that they were pregnant, as were a similar proportion of their partners.[1] This sometimes contrasted with the initially negative reactions of their friends and family:

> *My mother was faintly disgusted.*

> *You must be mad at your age . . . you are going to have an abortion.*

Don't you think you're a bit too old for this sort of thing?[1]

Workmates could also be insensitive:

> *The younger girls at work distance themselves from me. They've never given me their congratulations.*
>
> Betty, age 45, third baby, two grown-up children

However, very many women find that the people at work can also be important sources of support.

> *I'd like to talk to my mum but she's a worrier, and Jack* [partner] *has been in the army so he doesn't show his feelings, so I talk to one of the women at work, she's like a mum to me. I can ask her 'should I be feeling like this now?'*
>
> Marie, age 38 first pregnancy.

Entering the medical domain

Around one third of the women in the British study of 40-plus mothers were offered a termination.[1] Many were dismayed by this, particularly if it was offered when they visited their GP to confirm their pregnancy. However, nearly 40 per cent of the pregnancies in this study occurred in the 1960s and 1970s when medical attitudes to pregnancy after 40 may have been less favourable than they are today (1994), for reasons outlined in Chapter 5.

In the more recent Leicester Motherhood Project, where all the pregnancies occurred during the early 1990s, it was found that if older women did discuss termination this was usually in the context of antenatal screening (on around three quarters of occasions), and the discussion was usually expected, or initiated, by the woman herself (on two thirds of occasions).[2] Less than one third of women in their twenties said that anyone had mentioned the possibility of termination.

It is important to bear in mind the wide range of older women's individual experiences. For instance, Ruth, who conceived by IVF (in-vitro fertilization or 'test-tube' conception) at the age of 36, after 12 years of infertility treatment, felt *'somewhat miffed'* at her GP's reaction to her pregnancy:

> *I was deflated. He said I shouldn't count my chickens before they were hatched and emphasized the negative side ... wait till 20 weeks ... so I went out and bought some things for the baby straight away just to prove him wrong! He was fine at the next visit though.*

Ruth also found it hard to cope with the contrast between the intensive (and extremely supportive) monitoring she received at the NHS infertility clinic, and the level of monitoring provided during normal antenatal care. Having known that she was pregnant from an extremely early stage (almost immediately after conception) she found the long gaps between check-ups very hard to bear and would have welcomed more frequent reassurance that everything was proceeding normally, including more frequent ultrasound scans.

At the opposite extreme was Betty who became pregnant through contraceptive failure at the age of 45 when she and her husband were just starting to look forward to enjoying their new-found freedom from the responsibilities of parenthood now that their two children had grown up. At her mid-pregnancy interview she said:

> *My GP was almost reluctant to give me the 'morning after' pill because he said there was probably no need for it at my age ... I'd be very unlikely to conceive. But in the end he gave it to me ... I was really devastated and upset to discover that I was pregnant despite the pill, but when I finally went back to the doctor at 11 weeks he was really helpful.*

ॐ

Antenatal screening: bane or boon?

Despite enormous variety in the circumstances of women over 35, there is one feature of pregnancy which they tend to share, and that is an awareness of the fact that the chances of having a baby with Down's syndrome increase with age.[3,4]

Before continuing, we must point out that antenatal screening presents little or no worry to some expectant mothers for a variety of reasons to do with religious belief, or their own personal beliefs in their ability to cope, or because they feel, usually rightly, that their chances of having an abnormal baby are so small that there is no need to worry.

However, others feel very differently. They may not be prepared to terminate the pregnancy but nevertheless want early warning about any condition that might affect their baby. From the professional point of view the consensus now emerging is that it is unacceptable to make the offer of prenatal diagnosis conditional upon the prospective parents' agreement to abort an affected foetus.[5] Many women find screening and diagnosis extremely valuable:

> *The staff made a special effort to discuss things because of my age. I didn't want the blood test* [for Down's syndrome] *because it wouldn't give me the information I wanted, just a probability level but nothing about my particular baby, I'd be left in limbo: so I had the amnio . . . I was anxious for the whole of the four weeks* [i.e. waiting for the results] *. . . everything else had gone wrong this year so I thought this would be the last thing . . . but once I got the results it was really reassuring. I'd say women should take the tests – so you have less worrying time up to birth.*
>
> Maureen, 41, first baby

The actual probabilities of Down's syndrome and other conditions affecting the unborn baby are discussed in Chapter 5. In the rest of this section we shall focus on what it is like to be on the receiving end of the procedures which screen for these conditions.

We feel that the importance of this issue cannot be underestimated because, as we write, tests are beginning to be offered to all pregnant women which have formerly been available only to older women (or to younger women with a raised chance of having a baby with a detectable congenital abnormality). Obstetricians and the expectant parents who are their clients may agree that antenatal screening and diagnosis are important, but they may do so from different perspectives and therefore end up being at cross purposes with one another. Obstetricians may emphasize the potential reassurance associated with screening, and research suggests that parents may also welcome the new technology.[6] However, for expectant parents being faced with numerical probabilities of having a baby with Down's syndrome, and the potential option of terminating an affected foetus should amniocentesis give a 'positive' (but for the parents, a very negative) diagnosis, the whole character of pregnancy is altered. As one anthropologist suggested, the new technology introduces a new role for parents as 'quality controllers' on a genetic production line, with all the anxiety that this entails.[7,8]

How is information presented?

If an older woman attends a consultation with an obstetrician about antenatal screening or diagnosis, what information does she receive? One study suggests that the single most important determinant of ethical decision-making, within professional geneticists (this does not include obstetricians), is whether the geneticist is male or female: 'Women were less directive and more observant of patient autonomy than men.'[9]

In 1993 a group of British researchers reported their findings after tape-recording consultations about amniocentesis (*see Chapter 5*), with permission.[10] During *every* consultation, they found that obstetricians made an implicit assumption that women *should* have an amniocentesis, and that the word 'risk' was used, rather than a word without negative connotations such as 'chance', 'likelihood', or 'probability'. At *most* but not all consultations numerical probabilities (of abnormality or of miscarriage following amniocentesis) were presented (e.g. one in 100). However, these were often translated in a binary fashion by the obstetrician. In other words s/he tended to say whether the risk was high or low. This may have been done in an attempt to simplify complex information, but whether a probability level is *perceived* as high or low by the expectant parents may depend on many factors. Furthermore, probabilities given for the occurrence of Down's syndrome at a particular age and for the occurrence of miscarriage varied and were therefore sometimes inaccurate. The probability of miscarriage associated with amniocentesis tended to be described as low, but the *same* level of probability, if referring to chances of having a baby with Down's syndrome, was described as high.

The study, in common with others, revealed that doctors tend to underestimate how much information women wanted.[11] This may have arisen out of concern that too much information might provoke anxiety, but in fact relevant research has shown that extra information either has no effect on anxiety or reduces it.[12] They also tended to underestimate women's ability to understand information.

Only relatively rarely was it mentioned that amniocentesis could detect conditions other than Down's syndrome or that amniocentesis does not screen for all possible abnormalities. In fact 50 per cent of abnormalities detected by amniocentesis are conditions other than Down's syndrome; some have only very mild symptoms.[13] One report says that 'routinely available prenatal tests test for fewer than 50 per cent of serious birth abnormalities.'[11] None of the obstetricians described Down's syndrome or any of the other conditions detected by amniocentesis, neither did they ever mention that the test occasionally needs to be repeated if cells cannot be cultured from the sample of fluid obtained.

Maternal serum screening: Down's syndrome blood tests

The pregnant women in the consultations described above were trying to decide whether or not to have an amniocentesis on the basis of general information which applied to all women in their age group, not just to themselves. However, this situation is changing because of the introduction of blood tests (Bart's test, double, triple or quadruple test, 'Down's syndrome test') which provide information which is much more personal. For example, a pregnant woman may now be told that her chances, based on information from her own blood, of having a Down's syndrome baby, are one in 80, whereas for most women of her age the chances are one in 800. What does she do? As a woman in this predicament said during a Dutch research project, *'that is ten times as much. Such a difference forces you to apply for further diagnostic tests.'*[6] In other words this woman felt she should have an amniocentesis despite the possibility (around one in 150 or 200) of miscarriage associated with the procedure.

Would this woman have felt differently if she had been told that her blood test showed that there was a 98.8 per cent chance that her baby did not have Down's syndrome, compared with a 99.9 per cent chance for the 'average' woman of her age? Possibly not, and yet the information is mathematically identical. Box 6.1 suggests various ways of expressing the same information.

The dilemma of amniocentesis

Women tend to be very concerned about the possibility of having a Down's syndrome baby: the very fact of being offered an amniocentesis on the basis of their own personal blood test results makes them feel that the possibility is one to be taken very seriously. They cannot ignore the risk, but at the same time are faced with a very difficult dilemma because of the chances of miscarriage after amniocentesis.

> *I knew the risk of miscarriage was about one in 150. So in my case, the risk (of having a Down's syndrome child) is smaller than the risk of having a miscarriage caused by amniocentesis. I just don't know what to make of it.*[6]

In this context it has been found that what counts is not so much the actual probability of having a Down's syndrome baby but the

LOOK ON THE BRIGHT SIDE (BOX 6.1)

People are not very good at using probabilistic information to help them make decisions. One study makes this clear: people who were told to imagine there was a 20 per cent chance that their baby *had* Down's syndrome were compared with a group who were told to imagine that there was an 80 per cent chance that their baby did *not* have Down's syndrome.[14] What happened?

More people from the first group than from the second group said they would have had an amniocentesis.

But both groups of people were in fact given the *same* information, numerically: saying that there is a 20 per cent chance that something *will* happen is the same as saying there is an 80 per cent chance that it will *not* happen.

It is therefore important that all those involved in decision-making should be able to express information positively as well as negatively – to look on the bright side. In the area of antenatal screening this means that it is important to know the chances that a baby will *not* be affected by a condition as well as the chances that he/she *will* be affected.

The following instructions may help those who feel uncomfortable about the calculations involved.

What if chances of having a Down's syndrome baby are expressed as 'one in something' (e.g. 'one in 300')?

In order to look on the bright side, and to put it very simply, subtract *one* from the value you have been given (300 in this case, so the answer is 299). The chances that the baby does *not* have Down's syndrome are 299 in 300.

To express this as a percentage do the following sum on a calculator:

Work out the original value minus one, then divide the answer by the original number itself, then multiply this answer by 100. This last answer gives the percentage chance that the baby is *not* affected by Down's syndrome.

For the example above: $(300 - 1)/300 \times 100 = 299/300 \times 100 = 99.7$ i.e. a 99.7 per cent chance that the baby is not affected (this is the same as a 0.3 per cent chance that the baby *is* affected).

BOTH THESE ARE IDENTICAL:
1 IN 300 CHANCE OF DOWN'S
99.7 PER CENT CHANCE THAT THE BABY
DOES NOT HAVE DOWN'S

way parents perceive and interpret this probability, which is influenced by the way the information is presented.[14] We are not really 'designed' to process probabilistic information objectively because, as Jean, aged 39, said at mid-pregnancy, '*although the risk is only one per cent it's still a 100 per cent worry to the mother.*'

Cultural background is another factor that influences whether or not couples decide to risk amniocentesis. For instance in the US there is evidence that Jews tend to feel that amniocentesis is a humane addition to the resources available, but Haitian immigrants tend to reject it because they do not recognize Down's syndrome as a problem; there being no word for the condition in Creole.[7] The symptoms are not noticeable as a distinct syndrome in their country of origin where infant mortality is 50 per cent. As one Haitian father said:

> *The counsellor says the baby could be born retarded. They always say Haitian children are retarded. What is this retarded?*[7]

For those who do opt for amniocentesis, what does it feel like? Box 6.2 describes women's responses to this question.

Chorionic villus sampling (CVS)

This is a procedure described in Chapter 5 which allows for earlier diagnosis than does amniocentesis but carries with it a slightly higher probability of miscarriage (see, for example, Janine in Chapter 1). Research suggests that CVS is often seen as the preferred option by older, better educated women who have had few previous pregnancies or births, who are particularly likely to cope with situations by seeking as much information as possible.[5, 15] They feel that the advantage of knowing about abnormalities before they have felt the baby move or have had time to start feeling or looking pregnant outweighs the disadvantage of the higher likelihood of miscarriage.

WHAT DOES AMNIOCENTESIS FEEL LIKE? (BOX 6.2)

The quotes below are from women over 35 who received amnio-centesis in 1991 and 1992:

Not painful – the feeling you get when you shiver all over when 'someone walks over your grave'. Was told to take it very easy for the next 48 hours. Was told if I got to the weekend (six days) I'd probably be OK – not miscarry. I don't know what the percentage of miscarriage is with amnios but I feel that it is stressed very strongly that there is a big risk which makes it a very 'frightening thought'. I found the actual test a bit of an anticlimax.

Clair, 41, second baby, waited five weeks for results

Slightly uncomfortable, more painful afterwards than I expected . . . I was told to rest for at least 24 hours and not to go to work. However, I was not told about some of the other symptoms like pain where needle was inserted. Could be worrying – knowing there is a chance of miscarriage.

Janice, 36, first baby, waited four weeks for results

It was uncomfortable. I was told to sit down for half an hour immediately afterwards and to stay at home from work for 48 hours . . . I felt as though my body was in a state of slight shock for a couple of days after the amnio-centesis.

Betty, 45, third baby, waited three and a half weeks for results

It wasn't uncomfortable. I felt a slight, sharpish pain as the needle went through . . . was told to rest for half an hour afterwards, not to drive or walk home, to rest at home for 48 hours, to take things carefully there-after – for a few weeks but especially so in the first fortnight. I cancelled a plane trip to relatives abroad.

Angela, 35, first baby, waited four weeks for results

Just a little uncomfortable but that is probably because I was frightened it was going to harm the baby. I was told not to do any lifting, cooking, but just to put my feet up and rest for at least 24 hours.

Nagina, 36, waited six weeks for results

A strange sensation, not painful . . . Very good idea for older women. I may not have tried to conceive if it was not available.

Winnie, 40, second baby, waited four weeks for results.

The future of antenatal screening

The technological advances in antenatal screening are happening so quickly that the information we have presented here will need updating relatively soon. Research pinpoints the potential for both reassurance and anxiety associated with antenatal screening for Down's syndrome and other anomalies.[8] Although there is some evidence that many women feel screening is useful, there is evidence from a survey carried out in 1992 that as many as 40 per cent of midwives do not feel confident about counselling women undergoing serum screening and nearly as many do not feel termination of pregnancy for Down's syndrome is justified.[16] About one quarter were not in favour of serum screening for Down's syndrome.

Obstetricians, too, may feel ambivalent about some aspects of antenatal screening for Down's syndrome and about counselling: they receive no formal training in how to undertake this daunting responsibility.[10] Thus medical professionals and expectant parents alike are well aware of the practical and ethical dilemmas posed by antenatal screening and diagnosis. Research is now beginning to address these dilemmas, and there is a continuing and increasing need for it to do so as more procedures become available to wider groups of women.

ॐ
Worries in 35-plus pregnancy

The preceding section painted mid-pregnancy as a time of potential anxiety so far as antenatal screening and diagnosis are concerned. How does this one aspect of pregnancy fit into the wider picture?

The first possible source of concern for pregnant women of any age is whether the baby is all right. In the Leicester Motherhood Project mid-pregnancy was a time when older women worried more than younger ones about this issue and the possibility of miscarriage.[2] Although older women were more

---

MAKING SCREENING MORE POSITIVE (BOX 6.3)

Neutral words such as 'chance', 'probability' and 'likelihood' are preferable to the word 'risk' with its negative connotations.

Information produces different responses depending upon whether it is framed negatively (e.g. a 20 per cent chance of abnormality) or positively (e.g. an 80 per cent chance of *not* being affected).

Women find it helpful to discuss the implications of diagnostic test results *before* undergoing the tests, particularly if they perceive themselves as being at 'high risk'.[52] Extra information is extremely unlikely to cause extra anxiety and it may lessen anxiety.

All those involved – obstetricians, midwives, and parents and their families – need more support.

Parents who opt for termination following a 'positive' diagnosis may feel extremely isolated, more than those who experience other reproductive bereavements such as miscarriage or stillbirth. To date there is at least one support group for those concerned: SATFA.[52]

If Down's syndrome or another condition is diagnosed, termination is not the only option. It would help to ensure that expectant parents have access to support groups who can discuss the condition with them; perhaps enabling them to meet a child or adult with the condition, to enable decisions to be well-informed.

Detailed ultasound can help couples with a diagnosis of chromosomal abnormality to decide whether or not to terminate. Seeing a baby on ultrasound is more useful than seeing a description on paper such as 'de novo 13:22 translocation' or 'inherited (maternal) paracentric inversion of chromosome X'.

For older women the high level of anxiety provoked by antenatal testing in mid-pregnancy may be offset by very positive experiences of later pregnancy for the vast majority whose test results are reassuring.

---

anxious about the *results* of antenatal tests than were younger women (none of the younger women had an amniocentesis) older women were not more likely to worry about the *process* of having tests. For women of 35-plus who were expecting their second, third or fourth child, over 60 per cent said at mid-pregnancy that they thought life was going to be a lot more difficult after the baby arrived. First-time mothers were less likely to say this. In fact this reflected a realistic appraisal of the situation: after birth, 80 per cent of 35-plus experienced mothers said life was at least a little more difficult (compared with 65 per cent of first-time 35-plus mothers, and 73 per cent of those in their twenties). However, only 17 per cent of experienced mothers said it was *more difficult than they had expected*. Another study found that 30–39 year-old women expecting their first baby were more anxious about becoming a mother than 20–29 year olds.[17]

Pregnant women over a wide range of ages have more hypochondriacal beliefs than non-pregnant women, such as disbelieving a doctor's diagnosis of a mild condition thinking it is something more severe, or believing that they have contracted a new disease despite reassurances that they have not.[18] These fears are remarkably persistent throughout pregnancy so although they may contribute to a woman's fears for the safety of her foetus they do not explain this latter fear, which tends to lessen as pregnancy progresses.

What effects does worry have?

Some women, and health professionals, may wonder whether anxiety and stress can have long-term adverse effects on a developing baby. As Chapter 7 makes clear, research which has looked at age and overall levels of anxiety (not specific anxieties related to screening) suggests that older women may be less likely than younger women to be highly anxious.[19]

A foetus's heart rate can be affected, but not so as to endanger life, when its mother is upset or anxious.[20] This should not give cause for concern as it is completely normal for foetal heart rate to alter as a response to something that the baby notices such as a sound or bright light. Foetal behaviour can be altered by emotions such as those experienced when listening to music, and also by the reassurance the mother feels when she sees the baby on an ultrasound screen:[21] women who could see their babies on the screen and had parts of the anatomy pointed out to them became less anxious, and their babies less active, than mothers and babies who were undergoing scanning but were not shown the picture.

Severe emotional stress (in the mother) can make a foetus suddenly much more active than usual.[20] In 1980 doctors carried out ultrasound examinations on 28 panic-stricken women during an earthquake in Southern Italy. The foetuses showed 'numerous, disordered and vigorous' movements, and the high level of activity lasted from two to eight hours. However we hope that this level of stress will not be experienced in most 35-plus pregnancies! Generally speaking, women who are less anxious by nature may have foetuses who are less active than those of women who are more anxious, but it is not known whether the anxiety causes the activity.[20] Interestingly, women's estimates of how active a foetus is may not reflect its actual level of activity as seen on ultrasound.[22]

Does anxiety in pregnancy affect the baby after it is born? Infants of women who are low in anxiety in pregnancy tend to cry less and are less changeable in their moods than infants of highly anxious women. Anxious women often describe their babies as more difficult than average, or more hungry, after birth.[20] However, this does not mean that women who are anxious and have difficult babies need to blame themselves for causing the difficulty: nobody has established whether there is a causal relationship here. Both factors could be caused by something else such as complications of pregnancy, or ill health, or they could both be genetically caused (infants with very high activity levels when in the womb continue to have high activity levels after birth, so this could just be part of their personal make-up), or, possibly, a *baby's* emotional state and level of activity could cause anxiety in the *mother*.

How to cope with worry

Women who have high levels of emotional support from their partners during pregnancy experience lower levels of anxiety, and this may also apply after the birth.[23] In the light of research it would seem sensible to suggest that pregnant women of 35 or more who do feel particularly worried should try to express their worries to someone who is in a position to understand – or at least to listen attentively and sympathetically.[24] Medical staff can help enormously by giving as much information as possible. Some older women may feel reassured that they are being treated as a 'special case' because of their age, but to others special treatment may have the opposite effect:

> *Doctors made me aware that I was quite old to be a mother. I would've liked to have been patted on the head and reassured that I was not a freak.*[25]
>
> Lesley, 39, describing her second pregnancy

At the moment older women and their partners are still in a minority of new parents. They are therefore unlikely to have much contact with other women undergoing the same types of screening, and therefore do not have access to a source of support normally available to expectant mothers; nor will their own mothers have had the same experiences. They thus rely extremely heavily on medical professionals at all levels as their only sources of information and formal or informal 'counselling', placing strain on already stretched resources. We hope that, as the proportion of women giving birth after 35 continues to rise, and antenatal screening becomes more commonplace among all age groups, women will become more likely to find allies among their peers and a wider understanding of the terrible dilemmas posed for some by screening. The knowledge that they have coped with anxiety before in their lives and survived the experience, coupled with research findings suggesting that older women feel more positive about most aspects of pregnancy and motherhood than younger women by late pregnancy, may help to tide them over the negative aspects of mid-pregnancy.[2]

ॐ

Emotional and physical changes during 35-plus pregnancy

Emotional well-being

Turning to other aspects of pregnancy, the outlook for older women tends to be rather positive. For instance among women of 35 or more, levels of depression during pregnancy are not likely to be raised, and may in fact be low, relative to women in their twenties.[2, 26, 27, 28] This bodes well for older women as there is a significant relationship between being depressed (or not) during pregnancy and being depressed (or not) *after* the birth.[29, 30] Chapter 8 looks in more detail at the issue of depression after birth.

For most women, pregnancy is a time of positive mental health, and it may well have less effect on moods than is commonly assumed, according to a review by Margaret Oates.[31] Some women may, however, notice that their moods are much more changeable and unpredictable than they were prior to pregnancy. Different stages of pregnancy have been associated with different symptoms: tearfulness and irritability in the first trimester, easily feeling guilty but otherwise well in the second trimester, easily moved to tears and socially withdrawn in the third trimester. Older women may be less distressed by other people's opinions and are less likely to suffer from irrational fears (phobias).[2, 28, 32] On the other hand older first-timers may be particularly likely to say that they have felt 'touchy or easily offended' during pregnancy.[2]

American researchers have found that pregnant women, regardless of age, tend to be relatively self-critical during the transition to parenthood.[29] However, this may be less of a problem for older first-time mothers, as Ramona Mercer found that older women (aged 30–42) were more flexible, more highly integrated, had more positive or adaptive personality traits and childrearing attitudes, and were more competent than younger mothers.[33]

Are older women more tired during pregnancy?

Popular mythology suggests that older women are likely to become more tired before (and after) they have a baby, compared with younger women. Is this really the case? We found that age made no difference to how tired women said they were at late pregnancy.[2] Just under half the women questioned said they were *'so exhausted life had been very difficult'* or *'very tired'*, regardless of their age. Maybe the conclusion to draw here is that extreme tiredness in pregnancy is normal, but those who are older may wish to explain it with reference to their age.

Body image

At least two studies report that later childbearers experience little or no bother with physical symptoms and changes in their appearance.[32, 34] These findings are supported by our research in which older women were questioned about physical symptoms.[1, 2] It was found that although older women notice changes in their bodies and appearance they tend to find them less bothersome than younger women, particularly if they are expecting their first baby. The physical changes that most often caused 'bother' in the British study of 40-plus mothers tended to be heartburn, followed by bladder control, feet and ankle swelling, and back pain (experienced by around one third of women). We also found that older women report *fewer* symptoms such as nausea, breathlessness, dizziness and so on than younger women, during pregnancy.[2]

Cognitive changes: do pregnant women think straight?

Some women feel that they cannot concentrate very well, forget words, cannot think as rationally as usual, or do irrational things during pregnancy. Obviously all these abilities form an important part of problem-solving and may therefore have far reaching implications at a time such as pregnancy when women are faced with considerable life changes. They also influence the chances of accidents occurring.[35]

Some researchers suggest that pregnant women have some difficulty 'planning ahead'. Other researchers have linked changes in the way one thinks during pregnancy with nutritional deficits, suggesting, for example, that iron supplementation may improve some sorts of cognitive performance.[36] Other researchers suggest that it may be stress, rather than pregnancy per se, that affects thinking.

An Australian study found that over 50 per cent of women report general changes when pregnant such as memory problems, lack of concentration and attention, and increased absent-mindedness.[37] Women who were older, married or cohabiting, had a high level of education and were attending an obstetrician were likely to report more changes (77 per cent of women over 26, 44 per cent of women under 26). This is possibly because these women were involved in occupations in which cognitive changes 'showed up' more than they would do in less intellectual occupations, and possibly because older women are more adept at evaluating themselves and hence identifying and labelling the changes. Whatever the explanation, it is important for medical professionals and pregnant women alike to know that cognitive changes in pregnancy are normal and are therefore not the woman's 'fault' and need not result in self-blame and lowered self-esteem. Indeed, the higher rate of perceived cognitive change among older women may reflect high levels of self-awareness and hence, potentially, high levels of ability to cope with the changes of pregnancy.

Sexuality during pregnancy

Research into this topic is singularly thin on the ground. A recent survey of sexual behaviour in Britain contains not a single reference to sexual feelings or behaviour during pregnancy, neither did Kinsey's famous study of 8000 women.[38, 39] It is known that there are some relatively rare medical conditions in which intercourse and/or non-coital orgasm should be avoided, according to Kenneth Reamy and Susan White, among which are cervical incompetence, threatened miscarriage, repeated miscarriage with unknown cause, placenta praevia, and threatened premature labour.[40] Such conditions aside, there follows a summary of some findings, mostly to do with behaviours rather than feelings, with the proviso that there is very little scientific data on the subject.[41]

Most of the empirical information available to date on sex-related issues in regard to pregnant women and their foetuses is either inconclusive or contradictory.[40]

As an illustration of the contradictory nature of the advice given to pregnant women, one authority suggested that women who do not experience 'the release of orgasm' may be likely to deliver prematurely, whereas others have said as recently as 25 years ago that maternal orgasm will cause oxygen deprivation and lead to mental retardation in the baby. Neither of these suggestions has been found to hold true.[40] Maternal orgasm does tend to make the baby's heart-rate alter slightly but certainly no more and probably much less than the alterations the baby is 'designed' to cope with during normal labour. Orgasm and intercourse can cause strongly felt uterine contractions, especially in the third trimester,[41] but it has never been proven that maternal orgasm, or penetration without orgasm, leads to *premature* labour. Similarly, orgasm and/or penetration are unlikely to cause miscarriage: according to a review of research by Kenneth Reamy and Susan White, the vast majority of miscarriages are due to chromosomal defects and 'miscarriage due to trauma, injury, or physical activity is rare'. A foetus is very well protected from any impact during intercourse because the uterus is located deep inside the body and amniotic fluid is an extremely effective cushion.

Despite this, many women and/or their partners do feel concerned that sexual activity during pregnancy might affect the baby. Level of worry seems little affected by age but more 'first-timers' than 'experienced' mothers tend to worry about this.[2] Interestingly none have ever been reported to have felt worried that *lack* of sexual activity might have an adverse effect on the baby!

Some medical articles report that sexual interest and frequency of intercourse tend to decrease as pregnancy progresses, and that this must be universal as it has been reported in America, Thailand and the UK.[41] Others say that loss of interest in sex is common in the first trimester.[40] Still others say that it is impossible to predict changes in sexuality during pregnancy.[42] There does, however, seem to be agreement that women who are sexually experienced and enjoy the sexual side of their relationship will continue to do so during pregnancy, making any necessary adjustments such as using a 'side-by-side' position as their girth increases. Those who do not particularly enjoy sex before pregnancy are not likely to find that pregnancy alters this state of affairs, according to researchers; also, those who are depressed are likely to feel little interest in sex.

For some women who have been trying to conceive for years, pregnancy may present a welcome relief from seeing sex as a duty to be performed at the optimum time in the menstrual cycle and give them freedom to enjoy it if they wish.

> *Having waited for ten years to conceive it was a relief not to have to think whether 'this time' I'd get pregnant!*
>
> Ann, 37

Women of 35-plus expecting their first baby may be more likely than older women with children, or women in their twenties with or without children, to say that they often find their partner sexually desirable (80 per cent versus less than 50 per cent).[2] Older first-timers and younger pregnant women who already had a child were the groups who most often said that their partners found them desirable, but for the younger mothers this may have represented unwelcome attention as 43 per cent of them said that they did not look forward to sexual intercourse at all, compared with only a quarter of the other groups. More older (90 per cent) than younger (73 per cent) women seemed to find it easy to show affection to their partners, more older first-timers enjoyed kissing and petting, and more older women in general tended to feel easily sexually aroused.

Overall the picture that emerges from this research is that those expecting their first child, particularly those over 35, may feel more positive about sex and sexuality than do those who already have children. This may happen because, as one older woman with four children pointed out, having children around was the most effective contraceptive she knew because she and her partner had no time to themselves.

ॐ

Lifestyle and life changes in becoming an 'older mother'

Caffeine, nicotine and alcohol in midlife pregnancy

The harmful effects of cigarette smoking and alcohol during pregnancy are well-known. Caffeine consumption may also be of concern to pregnant women as some, but not all, research suggests that it may be associated with abnormalities.[43] A recent study showed that foetuses of women who drank a lot of coffee, tea, or other caffeinated beverages (more than 500 mg of caffeine per day) spent more of the time awake and active than did foetuses of women who consumed small amounts of caffeine.[44] (An 'average' cup of coffee contains about 100 mg of caffeine.) When they were born these babies weighed slightly less than the babies of women who drank less caffeine, and the researchers suggest that this was possibly because they spent more time in the womb in 'energy-consuming' activity. However, we have come across no research linking dangers of caffeine with maternal age.

In contrast, there is evidence that cutting down on smoking in pregnancy is even more beneficial to the babies of older mothers than it is for those of younger women, so far as preventing minor malformations is concerned.[45] These issues need sensitive handling:

If my consultant had just ordered me to stop smoking I'd have just turned against him and carried on. But he didn't . . . he made me feel that I was doing something really good to help my baby every time I didn't have a cigarette, and he really praised me for cutting down so that I ended up having just three a day, after meals and to relax in the evening.

Heather, 39, second child expected, conceived while taking fertility drugs

Sometimes pregnant women may take fewer healthy precautions, such as abstaining from smoking, than non-pregnant women because they feel so distressed about their belief that something is wrong with them that they do not feel it is relevant to take a long term view.[18]

However, smoking is not likely to be a problem characteristic of older pregnant women: there is evidence from the Children of the Nineties study that older women may smoke less than younger women during pregnancy, whereas looking at levels of alcohol consumption the opposite may apply, with older women tending to report slightly more drinking during pregnancy than younger women.[27]

Illegal drug use – are older women affected?

In one study which followed people from adolescence into mid-adulthood, Denise Kandel found that later marriage and child-bearing (or childlessness) were sometimes associated with the use of illegal drugs such as marijuana.[46] It is notoriously difficult to obtain reliable figures as to how many women use illicit drugs during pregnancy. People prefer not to admit to such behaviours because of the potential repercussions of such an admission. A recent American study analysed the meconium of new-borns in Detroit and found that around 44 per cent of them had been exposed to cocaine, opiates, or cannabinoids, or a combination of these, during pregnancy.[47] However, if they had relied instead on the mothers' reporting of drug use, only 11 per cent of the total sample would have been identified as having used drugs. This study found that there *was* a slight tendency for those with serious drug problems to be older, but also to be single, less well-off, to have had many previous pregnancies and to have had no antenatal care. Such high prevalence rates may be a reflection of the area in which data were collected. For instance, the Children of the Nineties study looked at cannabis use and found that very few women of any age reported it during pregnancy.[27] Any conclusions drawn here should be treated with caution because of the possibility that some who used the drug did not report it, but in early pregnancy women between 25 and 35 seemed least likely to have been users. Those of 35-plus were next (around one in 50), with those under 25 being most likely (around one in 21).

Findings relating to the effects of particular drugs on foetal development are scarce, because most researchers find that women who have used one drug tend to have used others, including tobacco and alcohol, and also to have other 'lifestyle' problems. Medical authorities agree, however, that any unnecessary drugs should be avoided in pregnancy, wherever possible.

Control over the baby's health

Given the level of concern that older pregnant women feel about whether their baby will be born healthy and normal, do they have different beliefs to younger women about the extent to which their baby's well-being is 'taken out of their hands'? Do they feel there is less, or more, that they can do themselves to give their babies the best chances possible?

Pregnant women who feel that they have plenty of control over their pregnancy and birth tend to be less likely to use street drugs, non-prescription drugs such as aspirin, and cigarettes.[48] In other words, those who believe they can influence their baby's health at birth take better care of themselves and their foetuses. Raised maternal age may have no effect on how much control women feel they have, although research in Poland found that older women had higher levels of belief in their own influence over foetal health.[48, 49] Older women in the Leicester Motherhood Project tended to be more likely than those in their twenties to say that 'chance' had a role in determining their baby's health at late pregnancy, but despite the fact that older women had more contact with medical professionals both they and younger women felt equally that doctors, midwives and nurses were rather unlikely to affect their baby's chances, and that they themselves were more important influences.

Believing in the baby

As recently as 50 years ago women would not have publicly acknowledged their pregnancies, or even have been completely sure that they were pregnant, until they were safely past the 'three-month hurdle' – past the stage at which miscarriage is most likely. With the advances in pregnancy testing, women are now able to determine whether or not they are pregnant at a very early stage. This has interesting implications, particularly for those over 35.

Early diagnosis of pregnancy is desirable in many ways as it lessens the suspense of wondering 'Am I or aren't I pregnant?', and gives women a chance to change drinking, smoking, or other lifestyle habits very early on in pregnancy, if they so wish. But what effects do early diagnosis of pregnancy have if women are to be offered antenatal screening which carries with it the possibility of termination of pregnancy? Even though the vast majority of women will find that the results of screening give them reassurance, older women in particular may intentionally try to distance themselves from their baby until the all-clear is given, possibly as late as 25 weeks into pregnancy if they have an amniocentesis.[50, 51] Older women may therefore have as long as five months of a 'limbo' state, and it is very difficult to remain detached from a foetus whose movements have been felt and who has been seen on ultrasound scans. In our study we found that around 75 per cent of first-timers, and 40 per cent of experienced mothers, felt differently about the baby after they had felt it move, regardless of their age. This happened between 13–24 weeks for first-timers (mean 19 weeks) and between 12–22 weeks for those expecting second or subsequent babies (mean 16 weeks).

Although older women, compared with younger ones, do tend to try not to get too attached to their foetuses at an early stage, they do not deny its existence to the extent of doing things that might harm it.[51] So does the deferral of attachment matter? This question is still being investigated and is assuming more importance as the screening giving rise to this 'tentativeness' is increasingly offered to younger as well as older women.

Some researchers have found that levels of attachment to the foetus during pregnancy are reflected in the mother–baby relationship after birth,[50] but other work suggests that women who have undergone screening 'catch up' with those who have not, in terms of adjustment and attachment, by late pregnancy.[2] Judging from research available we are therefore inclined to think that any effects of postponing belief in the baby are likely to be negligible and short-lived, relatively speaking, and need not give undue cause for concern.

⁊

What do older mothers wish they had known?

To conclude this chapter we shall pass on comments made by women of 35-plus during the Leicester Motherhood Project, as to what they wished they had known during pregnancy. Comments relating specifically to birth appear in Chapter 8. This is not advice backed up by academic research, but it is informed by first-hand experience.

Some women felt unprepared in different ways:

> *I wasn't prepared for the agony of breastfeeding . . . the fact that a large proportion of people I spoke to experienced sore, cracked and bleeding nipples and so many gave up. It is no wonder only 60 per cent breastfeed! The pain when the baby latches on does not subside for two to six weeks!*
>
> Suzanne, 36, first baby

New babies do not *sleep very much. Breastfeeding is painful long after cracked nipples have healed.*

Nina, 35, first baby

How uncomfortable and tiring it is [i.e. during pregnancy] *before the baby 'drops'. How sore and ill you can feel on the third day when your milk comes down. How tired you can feel after first taking your baby home with the broken nights.*

Gillian, 37, first baby

How easy it is to breastfeed. How enjoyable breastfeeding is; you really can almost see the bond.

Kate, 30, third baby

The change in your life is enormous. You can never 'go back'. The commitment is total, the work unending. But the love experienced was the deepest and most remarkable emotion in my life.

Lesley, 39, second baby

Before I had my first child I was not prepared for the enormous mood swings and terrible fears that occur after a few weeks of having a baby. I am a little more prepared for them this time around, even so, it is very disconcerting.

Andrea, 35, third baby

I found the first few weeks of sleepless nights and constant care very demanding and quite a shock. I think antenatal classes could do more on alerting expectant mothers to the changes they'll experience after the birth. The demands of a new baby, together with the physical problems associated with healing stitches and the major mood swings could be discussed in classes. Of course, until you've been through the experience it could be argued that you wouldn't understand the issues raised. However, talking about them beforehand could help to reassure a new mother that what is happening to her is quite 'normal'.

Beryl, 38, first baby

What advice would women pass on to others?

When breastfeeding in public always wear separates. It is much more discreet just to lift a jumper than to start unbuttoning. It looks as though you are just cuddling your baby.

Alison, 39, second baby

Even if breastfeeding is hard in the first week – hang on – it will soon be much better and worth it for both of you. Talk to other mothers about it for emotional support.

Deborah, 40, second baby

Having a baby completely changes your life and for the first few weeks (in my case) it is hard to do anything other than feed and look after the baby. Try and accept this situation because it does get better. In every other sphere of work people are trained to do the job in hand. You have no training in being a parent and that's what makes it so hard. Try and ignore people's advice unless you have asked for it – because everyone but you – it seems – is an expert. Do always ask for help from anyone available, for example, midwife, health visitor, doctor – that is what they are there for. Try and make a habit of getting out by yourself and with your husband, otherwise things can stagnate.

Suzanne, 36, first baby

The most important thing a mother should remember is that the love she feels for her child should never be denied or treated as 'spoiling' – we are too often made to feel inhibited about our normal protective and loving behaviour – sometimes to the detriment of children's upbringing.

Andrea, 35, third baby

Accept as much help as possible before and after birth. Turn a 'blind eye' if things are not done the way you would prefer.

Dawn, 43, first baby

Enjoy the first few weeks with your new baby. Don't want him/her to grow up too quickly. Take as much time as you can to just hold and love your baby – the time will soon pass and leaves a lovely memory. Your baby wants to love and please you – sometimes this is hard to remember after successive nights of non-stop colic! Don't torture yourself if you do shout or scold your baby. It is soon forgotten by both of you.

There is nothing wrong with having a baby in bed with you. It makes night feeds much easier and after a fraught, broken night, all can be forgiven and forgotten when you wake up to baby nestled beside you.

If you have pets, be patient – you will like them again. They are very forgiving and willing to please as well.

Nina, 35, first baby

Accept all help offered postnatally. Do your pelvic floor exercises. Enjoy the labour. Follow your instincts – I find this difficult but when I don't, with hindsight, it would have been better if I had.

Isabel, 35, first baby

Make sure that you are very much at ease in your relationship with your husband/partner because even the most well adjusted can be tried by the arrival of a baby.

Alison, 39, second baby

Try to find a little space for yourself particularly when the baby is born, even if it's to have a long bath, going to the shops etc . . . Enjoy the time before birth with your partner, and discuss both your thoughts and feelings fully.

No matter what, hold on to a sense of humour and don't forget you're not alone.

Don't feel guilty or uptight – find out what feels right for you, your baby and partner, and as long as you're all comfortable, thriving and happy, it's okay – don't, above all, be swamped by advice, information – sift through and only use what you find helpful and don't worry if your pregnancy, feelings, birth etc . . . aren't text book or how you think others react/cope/feel. Above all, I'd say relax, enjoy your pregnancy, the birth of your child, and its first few months; they all go by so quickly.

Gillian, 37, first baby

✎ 7 ✎

Self and Others: the Mother's Social World

Because my moods are up and down I need more support now than
before I was pregnant, but my family all understand ... my partner,
the midwife, my children, all help. They're really good.

Sharon, 37, pregnant with fourth baby,
three children from previous relationship

When a new baby is on the way, can the support of friends and
family make a big difference to an older mother? As described in
Chapter 6, pregnancy at any age is often seen as a time of
emotional and mental disturbance. For example, Lesley,
expecting her second child at the age of 39, wrote during late
pregnancy:

I keep feeling I want to be thrown a lifeline or rescued, especially when
my existing child is demanding a lot of attention. I would love to be
pampered.

These disturbances are so common that they can be described as
perfectly normal; creating and giving birth to a new human being
is an awesome and wonderful prospect which involves emotional
adjustment and physiological upheaval. Pregnancy can be a time
when priorities change and perspectives shift. With this in mind,
what effects can family, friends, and others have on adjustment to
pregnancy? And what effects can pregnancy have on relationships with other people?

ℑ

Pregnancy: setting the pattern for parenthood

In the short term, the way a woman feels about her relationships has a day-to-day influence on her moods. In addition, pregnancy represents just the first stage of a life-long process of adjusting to being the mother of the particular person she is carrying. There is plenty of evidence, discussed later in this chapter, indicating that a woman's 'psychosocial environment' – her relationships with other people in general – during (and before) pregnancy can influence how contented and well-adjusted she and her family are, even three years after the baby is born. Research also shows that a woman's psychosocial environment can have an impact on how healthy her new baby is.

The specific ways in which a person's psychosocial environment affects them depends partly on what that person is like. Some women welcome plenty of contact with friends and family; others may actively avoid too much social contact during pregnancy:

> *I've felt I wanted to avoid arguments and disagreements especially with my partner. I've felt distant from friends and relatives, lazy about keeping contacts up.*
>
> Andrea, 35, expecting third child

Are pregnant women of 35-plus likely to feel better supported and more secure than younger women? This chapter starts by examining how the individual characteristics and circumstances of women over 35 may be different from those of younger pregnant women, and hence how their experiences of their psychosocial environments may differ. However, as we made clear in Chapter 1 there are, of course, many differences *among* women of 35-plus: just because they belong to the same age-group does not mean that they share everything in common.

ॐ

Do people create their own social worlds?

Pregnant women are not passive recipients of things people say to them and expect of them. Much research suggests that women who have reached the age of 35 are likely to have psychosocial environments which differ in some ways from those of younger women, and this is partly of their own making. What evidence is there that someone's personality can affect their psychosocial environment? The next two paragraphs apply generally, but are of course relevant to women pregnant at 35-plus as well.

The role of personality in making and keeping friends.

It is known that some people have personality characteristics (they do, say, and feel things) that make it easy for them to make friends, and then to develop and maintain their friendships and enjoy them. This, in turn, seems to make it easy for them to obtain help when they really feel they need it.[1] So people's personalities can influence how much social support they have – how much they feel as if they belong, how happy they are with the quality of their relationships and how helpful they feel other people are.[1] One American reviewer points out that there are only a few scientific studies that look at both social support *and* personality, and that in the few that do consider both, social support seems relatively less important.[2]

The role of personality in feeling stressed

An Australian study that tracked people's lives through the 1980s found that the same or similar stressful things kept on happening to the same people.[3] The researchers said that each person has a pattern of stressful events that is normal for them (but might seem very stressful, or very stress-free, to someone else) and a pattern of subjective well-being is also normal *for them* and that both these patterns depend on that person's personality. In other words, people's personalities, the ways they habitually react to situations, actually determine – to some extent – what happens to them and how stressed or otherwise they feel when something happens.

$$\sim$$

'Time makes you bolder': true or false?

Is it really true that 'Time makes you bolder'?[4] Throughout a woman's life she has some choice concerning to whom she listens and whose opinions she values. In other words, as the preceding research examples suggest, we each have some control over our psychosocial environment, and play a part in creating it with every gesture and every word. Does this mean that by her mid-thirties a pregnant woman may be in an advantageous position, compared with somebody in her twenties, in that she has had time to find and/or form a 'niche' in which she is content with the company of those around her and can express herself to them without anxiety or fear? With a few exceptions there is little research into this issue, although psychologist Sheila Rossan says: *'If you look at the difference between a 20 year-old and a 35 year-old mother the whole mind-set is different.'*[5] There is some evidence to suggest that around mid-adulthood women become more concerned with their own identity and more self-confident and assertive than they were previously. This is at a time when men have been found to start to celebrate the importance of intimacy and personal relationships. As Carol Gilligan puts it:

> *The discovery now being celebrated by men in mid-life of the importance of intimacy, relationships and care is something women have known from the beginning.*[6]

(Male readers may prefer to rephrase this to describe women's discovery of confidence and assertiveness as something men have known all along!)

Other researchers argue that this phenomenon – the change in personal emphasis for women and men – is not restricted to western cultures. For example, in the cultures of both the Navaho Indians and the Lebanese, Western observers in the 1970s noticed that men tended to become more passive and contemplative as they grew older whereas women became more active, assertive and dominant.[7]

If women do feel more autonomy, confidence and a sense of identity in middle adulthood than they did in their twenties, is this just because of the passage of time? Or does it apply only if the woman has had children, watched them grow up, and started enjoying her new-found freedom? Some might argue that having children provides a learning experience that is completely unique. One study suggests that the purported increase in autonomy (feeling in control, able to make one's own decisions) may happen regardless of whether or not a woman has finished childbearing. Concluding her description of interviews with American women who gave birth after 35 in the early 1980s, Iris Kern said:

> Mothers interviewed, irrespective of race or social class, described themselves as having frequently done all they wished to do – travelled, accumulated material things, partied, achieved professionally and/or personally etc. *At this point in their lives they saw themselves as less competitive and more satisfied with their choices, with themselves, and with their babies.* (our emphasis)[8]

In the Leicester Motherhood Project, women who were pregnant were asked to say which words out of a list of adjectives described how they felt.[9] It was found that women of 35-plus were more likely than women in their twenties to describe themselves as feeling 'in control', although in fact only a minority of each age group chose this phrase (32 per cent of 35-plus women, 18 per cent of those in their twenties). Interestingly, however, it was only among 35-plus women that the phrase *'out of control'* was chosen (by 11 per cent) to describe how they felt at mid-pregnancy.

Other research comparing younger first-time Canadian mothers with those over 35 found that older women had a more autonomous personality style than younger ones.[10] Why might this be? Possibly, women born in the 1950s (i.e. the older group) are more autonomous than those born in the 1960s (the younger group). On the other hand it is possible that women who choose not to have children in their twenties are different in personality from those who do, and that this, not age alone, is the crucial explanation. There is research to support this idea.

The role of personality in the timing of parenthood

One study in particular suggests that personality may have a part in determining whether people become parents 'off-time'.[11] The findings of this study were that women who delayed parenthood (in this case to follow a career) scored just as high on measures of well-being as those who opted for 'normal time' motherhood, but they were less worried about norms and more able to resist constrictive pressures. Women who gave birth earlier in life found that motherhood brought with it an increase in responsibility, tolerance, and nurturance, but also led to a decrease in confidence and self esteem, and a suppression of impulse and spontaneity. The researchers found that some of these personality traits could be identified while the women were still in education: in other words, *before* starting their families.

Thus it is possible that pregnant women over 35 may differ at the outset from their younger counterparts. Particularly if parenthood has been delayed intentionally, a picture emerges of women who value their autonomy: although as pointed out in Chapter 3 there may be more difference between those who *never* have children and those who *delay* childbearing, than between 'off-time' and 'on-time' childbearers. Of course, the way 'off-time' parenthood is defined will vary from one decade, or one culture, to another.

However, no pregnant woman lives in a social vacuum: autonomy does not imply isolation. Indeed, two important aids to feeling autonomous are the existence of mutually satisfying, intimate relationships with others, and the feeling of being part of a wider society.[1] Therefore, the next step in the discussion is to look at how a pregnant woman's interactions with and feelings about others might affect her own well-being and that of her baby, starting with 'other people' in the broadest sense.

ی

Society and survival

Do older mothers encounter adverse reactions to their pregnancies because of their age? If they do, does this have any effects on their well-being or that of their babies and could it even affect their chances of being born at all? Of course the vast majority are born, but here we shall consider whether, in a very small percentage of unborn babies, society may make a crucial difference to the baby's survival, with particular reference to women over 35.

Abortion

Until 1981, women age 40 and over were more likely to have an abortion than to continue with a pregnancy, as was described in Chapter 2.[12] Why was this? There were probably many reasons, but one of them must have been to do with the way 'older motherhood' was perceived by society at that time. Older women may have felt that having a baby later in life was not a socially acceptable option. This is supported by a comment from one woman who gave birth to her third child, conceived accidentally after an eight year gap, in the 1960s, when she was 29:

> *I felt entirely out of place: of course I really was old by those standards, 29, nearly 30, in a ward of women in their late teens and early twenties.*[13]

If this feeling of alienation existed for those still in their twenties (and other accounts suggest that this was not an isolated instance) then it must have been even more marked for those in their late thirties or forties. Since 1981 the birth rate has exceeded the termination rate for women over 40, suggesting that social pressures may be changing.[12]

Suicide

A second somewhat stark topic is suicide. It is included here because it is an example of an event which can be influenced by a woman's relationships, and which rather obviously affects a baby's survival chances. Reassuringly, pregnant woman are *20 times less likely to commit suicide* than those who are not pregnant, even though pregnancy is a time when they may be prone to psychiatric disturbance. This was revealed by a count of *all* the suicides recorded in England and Wales between 1973 and 1984.[14] Only 14 suicides of pregnant women were reported in the 12 years, and *not one* pregnant woman of 35 or more committed suicide.

༫

Society in general:
are older mothers out of step?

Although older mothers are a fast-growing group, around 90 per cent of babies are born to women under 35 and this tends to be noticeable to many older mothers. Research has shown that it is less stressful to experience important life events such as starting a career, getting married, having children, or menopause, when these events happen at the socially expected times.[15, 16] An event that happens at an age deemed socially inappropriate is likely to be experienced as more stressful than it would have been had it happened at the 'normal' time. From this premise it could be argued that becoming a mother later in life must be stressful simply because most women who become mothers do so in their twenties. If this were true it would give cause for concern, because it has been suggested that *some* women (for example, those who are very poor, underweight, or in poor health) experiencing more stress during or before pregnancy may have less healthy babies.[15, 17, 18] Definitions of stress vary from one study to another but research tends to suggest that increased age, on its own, does *not* lead to higher levels of stress.

It is also well-established that, in general, low levels of stress make women less vulnerable to depression (and to other things such as psychosomatic symptoms and physical illness).[19] Depression rates during pregnancy may closely shadow rates after the birth.[20] This means a substantial number of women who do not feel depressed during pregnancy will not feel depressed after birth. So far as women over 35 are concerned, as with stress, research indicates that increased age alone does *not* appear to make women more likely to get depressed before or after childbirth, as mentioned in Chapter 6. There is thus no reason to suppose that 35-plus pregnant women as a group will suffer from being 'out of step', although of course individual circumstances will differ.

Finally, society's views of older mothers are constantly changing. There has been much recent (1995) media coverage of women who give birth in their fifties and sixties via egg donation. Women in their thirties and forties can thus be perceived as relatively young in some contexts.

ॐ

The need for social support

The discussion of other people so far has focused on society at large. Moving on from here, how do relationships with particular other people have an impact on the emotional and physical well-being of a pregnant woman?

Many researchers say that high levels of social support can 'cushion' the negative effects of stressful and unpleasant events.[21] However, others find that social support does not have this buffering effect.[15] This may be due to differences in the way 'social support' is defined and measured in different studies. It may also depend on who provides the support, and whether or not the support is perceived as helpful. So does social support matter?

Loneliness, social support and the health of older women

Having a feeling of belonging, of being part of the lives of others, gives a sense of 'social regulation':[1] it can provide an anchor of stability during times like pregnancy when things are changing very rapidly. However, change is not necessarily a negative thing – Angela had not felt ready for a baby until she was 35, and she commented on the unexpected joy of having things in common with other mothers:

> *It's quite amazing – as if there was a whole aspect of your life missing before ... so far as empathy with other women is concerned.*

People who lack a feeling of belonging tend to be somewhat oversensitive in that they exaggerate or misinterpret the hostility or the affection expressed by others; even everyday encounters with complete strangers may assume great importance. They are also more prone to medical problems such as headaches, poor appetite and feeling tired, as well as some serious illnesses.[22]

However, on the positive side, so far as older pregnant women are concerned, it was found in the Leicester Motherhood Project that age made no difference to whether or not women felt lonely during pregnancy.[9] Around three quarters of both age groups (twenties and 35-plus) said they 'never' or 'rarely' felt lonely.

The link between loneliness or friendship and health is important to mention here because healthier women are likely to have healthier babies. This is true regardless of age; at least one doctor has said that it is better (for mother and child) to be a healthy pregnant 38 year-old than an unhealthy pregnant 28 year-old.[23] Older women could be at an advantage in this respect given that most research finds that the 'average' older woman pregnant with her first child has spent more time in education and paid work than a younger woman (*see Chapter 2*), so has good housing and an adequate income: all factors which are associated with good health.[24] However, there is always the possibility that for some women the cause of their delay in childbearing is chronic illness.

Dwenda Gjerdingen agrees that social support has an immediate effect on mental health and a delayed effect on physical health.[24] She and her co-workers say that research shows that the changes in women's roles that accompany childbirth may have a negative effect on women's health in the short term, but that over the years combining the many roles associated with motherhood tends to be connected with having good health.

Health professionals

In the Leicester Motherhood Project women over 35 were more often classified as being of high medical 'risk status' at the start of their pregnancy than were women in their twenties, they had more ultrasound scans, and were more likely to be offered (and accept) amniocentesis.[9] The notion of whether or not a woman's pregnancy is regarded as being 'at risk' is an interesting one. Andrew Schuman and Theresa Marteau found that obstetricians tended to view pregnancy at any age as a state of risk, and the more experience they acquired the more they felt this, whereas midwives, however experienced, saw it as a 'normal' condition.[25] It is quite possible that this phenomenon might affect older women and younger women differently. Whatever the explanation, older women's experience of support from medical professionals differs from the experience of younger women, if only in terms of the number and nature of the contacts they have with them.

This age difference may apply from the instant a woman presents herself for medical inspection. In the British study of 40-plus women it was found that around one third reported having been offered a termination, often at the point at which they went for a pregnancy test. The majority of these women had their baby in the 1980s.[26]

More recent data suggest that in the 1990s women are not likely to be offered a termination on the grounds of age alone.[9] Where termination was discussed in the Leicester Motherhood Project it was usually in connection with screening for chromosomal abnormalities (*see Chapter 6*). Older women were slightly more likely than younger women to say that their GP had been helpful, or very helpful, on their first visit to her/him. Thus family doctors in the 1990s appear to show sensitivity to the needs of pregnant women of 35 or more.

What are the effects of professional support?

Some researchers and health professionals feel that professional support (for example from a midwife doing home visits) can reduce the chances of premature birth or of having a low birthweight baby. Findings so far indicate that such support, although it does not necessarily affect birthweight, does enhance women's sense of well-being and hence their ability to enjoy life, and that this effect is apparent even a year after the birth.[27, 28, 29] Lyn Quine and co-researchers summarize some of the beneficial effects of social support in pregnancy and labour thus:[30]

> *Fewer admissions to hospital during pregnancy; shorter labours; greater awareness during delivery; less use of neonatal intensive care by babies; greater health service use by mothers and babies after birth; and improved psychological well-being, especially a reduction in anxiety.*

Families and friends

> *All my family are a long way away, it's just down to my husband and he doesn't fully understand how I feel. Someone in my family would pre-empt my feelings, think ahead; he doesn't.*
>
> Tina, 39, expecting third baby

Dwenda Gjerdingen and colleagues reviewed existing research

and came to the conclusion that a partner's support is definitely important (see the last section of this chapter) so far as a woman's adjustment to becoming a mother is concerned, but that findings are inconclusive as regards the effects of other family members including parents and in-laws.[24] So what are the findings, in more detail?

In an American study pregnant women aged 14–38 were asked to say how satisfied they were with the support they were getting in various areas of their lives, and they were also asked to say whether anything stressful had happened in the year before their pregnancy.[15] The researchers reported that the *older* a woman was the *less* likely she was to be highly anxious. Age made no difference to whether or not women had high or low levels of support, but they did find that women who had higher levels of family support had babies with higher APGAR scores (*see Chapter 5*), and women who had experienced fewer stressful life events before their pregnancy had babies of higher birthweight.

Other studies have illustrated the complexity of the issue, even without trying to work out whether a mother's age makes a difference. Lyn Quine points out that socio-economic status is important, and Suzanne Cliver reported that women who were depressed, anxious, stressed, lacked self-esteem and a sense of control were likely to have babies who did not grow as quickly as they should while in the womb.[30,18] They were also more likely to have a low birthweight baby, but only if they (the mothers) were thinner than average. She was looking at a population of low-income black women in the US and argued that in *this* population, but not necessarily in others, being relatively heavy for your height will protect you from the adverse effects of being stressed and anxious.

Because of their increased level of education (*see Chapter 2*) and hence career aspirations, it might be predicted that 35-plus women are more geographically mobile than younger women. In other words they are relatively likely to live away from the area in which their parents live, so they may be more likely than younger women to rely on friends and partners for support than on their immediate family. This is true to some extent for mothers in an urban society regardless of age, as a comparison of women in Greece and the UK showed.[31,32]

ARE FAMILIES ALWAYS FRIENDLY?

It could be argued that friends have an advantage over family as a source of support: we have no choice over who is in our family but *can* choose friends. It has been shown that having access to a large family network does not necessarily lead to benefits in terms of the *health* of expectant mothers and new babies.[33] The Greek studies showed that a family network can be a source of stress, both during pregnancy and after the birth.[31, 32] This was also apparent in the Leicester Motherhood Project:[9]

> *I live with my mother-in-law. I didn't mind the amount of work before I was pregnant: all the housework is left to me – relatives come with their children and no-one else does anything. In our culture* [Hindi] *a woman is supposed to eat certain things at certain times in pregnancy; normally her mother looks after her. Mine doesn't and she didn't for my sister either although she lives near. I feel upset when I see my mother-in-law who does anything for her daughters but mine doesn't for me. So I shall refuse to go to my mother's after the baby is born, I'll look after myself.*
>
> Nagina, 36, first pregnancy

And after the baby was born:

> *My mother-in-law wants to give her* [the baby] *drugs from India to make her sleep so that I can get on with the housework. I won't give them to her. If she's awake and not being fed I have to give her to my mother-in-law so I can do the kitchen work. My mother-in-law and her daughter sit here and wait for me to finish with the baby so that I can do the cooking – they sit here doing nothing.*

To counter this, many older women comment on the way their maturity helps them deal with, or deflect, any interference from either friends or families. In the Leicester Motherhood Project only one quarter of first-time 35-plus women said they had felt bothered by people's comments, compared with over one half of the younger first-timers. Research evidence suggests that families and friends provide different sorts of support. Friends provide intimacy whereas families provide more practical help such as cleaning, cooking, shopping, or lending money.[19] In the Leicester Motherhood Project, more women over 35 than younger women felt in need of extra practical help after the birth, regardless of whether or not they had had children before. Thus older pregnant women might like to 'line up' potential volunteers to help with shopping, housework and so on, before the baby arrives. This age difference did not emerge so far as emotional support was concerned.

AGE OF THE FUTURE GRANDPARENTS

Does it matter that babies of older mothers may have very elderly grandparents? This question often crops up in media discussions of midlife mothering. Given that grandparents these days are not the only source of support for expectant and new parents we have to conclude that the answer is 'it depends ...'.[31,32] It depends on the individual circumstances of each family concerned. On the positive side, life expectancy is on the increase, and this implies that people may be healthier for longer. Today, grandparents aged 50 to 60 when their grandchildren are born can expect to live until their grandchildren are in their late teens at least, and because of the lower life expectancy in the past, grandparents who were only in their forties when their grandchildren arrived at the turn of the century could expect no more (figures are based on average life expectancies of those who survive childhood).[34] Indeed, one participant in the Leicester Motherhood Project pointed out a rather macabre advantage of having older parents and grandparents:[9]

> *They won't be dogged by elderly relatives for ages ... we'll die in time to give them some freedom*
>
>   *Deborah, 40 at the birth of her second child*

ADDING TO AN EXISTING FAMILY

So far there has been little mention of women in their late thirties or forties who already have children. In fact, the majority of babies born to women of this age will have older brothers or sisters (78 per cent of births to married 35-plus women in 1992 were to women who had previous live-born children).[35] Does pregnancy and the new arrival affect these women differently to first-time older mothers? They may worry that older sisters or brothers will find it hard to adapt, particularly if the new baby is the first fruit of a second marriage or partnership. As Jill said, looking back after the birth of her second daughter, Emma, at 35:

> *Zoe* [aged three at Emma's birth] *was tremendously jealous at first, there was a lot of regression, insisting on having a bottle and wearing a nappy and so on. Now* [six months] *she's fine, she's taken ownership of the baby. We knew we would have trouble because the baby was back home from hospital, with me, before we could collect Zoe from my mum's* [who lived a long distance away]. *It was unavoidable, the only way we could manage. We were right about having trouble, but we're OK now.*

Eileen's older children were 15, 14, 11, and 6 when Tom was born, and Eileen, herself, was 40. When she was asked how the children were coping she said:

> *They're all brilliant! It was the cats who were jealous, trying to get between me and the baby when she was feeding: but there was no viciousness, even from them.*

She explained that things had worked out better than expected:

> *I had wondered how it would affect Natalie* [aged six] *because there's a very close bond between me and her. I'm very glad the boys were older. I suppose in some ways Natalie got a bit of a bad deal, she had to grow up. It was a bit of a shock to the system for her, but not bad in the long term at all . . . I feel that all five of them are very close. Having Tom has strengthened that. It makes them all feel reasonably*

important, undertaking that role [of helping to care for Tom] *and knowing that they're being trusted to do it.*

Research evidence in this area, looking specifically at 35-plus women, is scanty. In the Leicester Motherhood Project in which levels of occupation and education were the same for older and younger women, older women who were expecting their second, third, fourth or fifth baby did comment on some difficulties to a greater extent than did first-time mothers of any age, or younger mothers who already had children.[9] For instance, when they were asked to choose from a list words or phrases that described themselves, descriptions such as 'angry', 'out of control', 'stressed', 'as if my body isn't my own', 'resentful', and 'vulnerable' were chosen more often by older experienced mothers than by any other group. However, positive descriptions such as 'happy', 'maternal', and 'in control' were also chosen most often by this group. Thus older experienced mothers display a wide range of feelings. On the negative side, Wendy, aged 36 at the birth of her second child said:

> *When you become a mother you get a label. I'm a housewife, John's wife, Robert and Lorna's mother . . . I'm not seen as an individual, I've become part of a package. Things I used to be able to do, I can't do now. You learn to expect less so you lose confidence. I don't wake up with a list of things to do any more.*

Or, more positively, Tina, having her third child at 40:

> *During the year since I had Sam I've felt I could cope with anything. We've had all sorts of mishaps, my husband's been rushed into hospital twice . . . When everything's been awful Sam's been wonderful, he takes the friction out of things.*

One study suggests that practical or material support (help with housework for instance) is particularly valuable to second-time prospective mothers, and that expectant parents wished that people would make fewer negative comments about whether it was wise to be having another child or remarks such as 'Haven't you had that baby yet?'[36] Although older women tend to be better able to cope with negative comments, it is clear than even if one has experienced pregnancy, birth and parenthood before, each new pregnancy brings a new set of challenges.[9]

OLDER MOTHERS LIVING ALONE

Statistics show that in 1992 nearly one in five women giving birth over 35 were opting for motherhood outside marriage.[35] However, it is likely that most of these were in a relationship with a partner with whom they lived: the only way of finding out is to look at whether the babies were registered by both parents and if so whether or not both parents gave the same address. In 1992, 2600 babies were born to 35-plus women who registered the birth in their own name only, and a further 2162 were born to parents who did not live together, although both were named on the birth register. Altogether, these births to lone mothers made up seven per cent of births to 35-plus women in 1992. Iris Kern reports that 12 per cent of her volunteer sample of American older mothers were unmarried at the time of her study and one woman summed up her view of single parenthood as follows:[8]

> *I sincerely believe single parenting is better than a less than ideal relationship. I wouldn't inflict a less than really good relationship on a child!*

This view is not always shared by the relatives of pregnant single women of this age, as is suggested by Angela's experience, recorded in Chapter 1.

Researchers have reported that *young*, unpartnered women can be at a disadvantage: for example more have been found to give birth to a baby with low APGAR score.[17] It is not known to what extent problems of this nature can be ascribed to the women's single status, to their youth, or to a complex combination of other drawbacks faced by young women in this situation. Because 35-plus women are typically at an advantage over younger ones in terms of earning potential and housing (*see Chapter 2*), findings pertaining to lone mothers in general may not be relevant for them.

In a study of 50 single Israeli women (unwed and not cohabiting) who gave birth when they were 30–45, Ruth Linn found that most of the women were not at a disadvantage socially.[37] Over 60 per cent did not have to find alternative housing because of the arrival of a child, 80 per cent had a stable profession. Although 64 per cent would have liked to marry given the right circumstances, 96 per cent said they would have done it again, and 90 per cent reported that pregnancy measured up to their expectations. The reactions of the people with whom they worked tended to be positive, and the women felt as if they had gained in professional competence because of the way in which their personal competence was boosted by having a child.

35-PLUS MOTHERHOOD IN A LESBIAN RELATIONSHIP

Of the seven per cent of women giving birth for the first time at 35-plus who do not live with the father of the baby, some will be in a lesbian relationship. Omission of any discussion of babies born to *lesbian women over 35* is a reflection of a lack of research on this topic. However, we feel that such babies must have been carefully considered and very much wanted in view of the impossibility of accidental pregnancy in such a relationship (barring rape etc). For instance, when asked in a questionnaire how 'wanting to be a mother' felt, Greta, aged 28, wrote:

> *I think it feels very, very different to think about, let alone go ahead with, choosing to have a child within a same-sex relationship. I believe I do have something like 'maternal urges', but these are very unpredictable and short-lived, and make me mistrust them. I have many confusing and contradictory feelings about it. Part of me believes I would be an excellent mother.*

When asked how she would feel if she discovered that she would never be able to bear a child:

As a lesbian there are numerous reasons and pressures for me not to have a child. But if it was a question of biology or physiology causing infertility, for example, then I might alternate between feeling cheated somehow, and philosophical and accepting of 'nature'. When sexual preference and the indulgence of it <u>doesn't</u> procreate, the whole question of choice and decision surrounding conception is raised (lesbians have wonderful imaginations). So I'm very torn – never to have children means a particular freedom, but only if it's a choice. And vice versa. I do believe in nature's aunts.

Such careful consideration augurs well for lesbian parents and their children as it has been established that adjustment before and after birth is better when a baby is wanted.[38] A Belgian reviewer points out that children brought up by homosexual couples following a separation or divorce do not have particular psychological, learning, or sexual difficulties, as they develop.[39]

OLDER MOTHERS WITH MALE PARTNERS

Where the prospective mother and father are married or cohabiting, how can their relationship with each other affect their baby? For that matter, how can having a baby affect the parents' relationship? Is there anything special older mothers should know? The rest of this chapter looks at the story so far revealed by research.

There are various ways in which other people can have an effect on the physical well-being of a baby during pregnancy. Straightforward physical injury is, of course, one way in which a developing foetus can be damaged. It has been argued that pregnant women are more likely than non-pregnant women to experience physical abuse from those close to them (e.g. husband or partner).[40] However, it has also been found that within marriage older men and women are less likely than younger ones to engage in physical aggression.[41] Therefore, although we have found no research linking violence in pregnancy with maternal age, it seems possible that older pregnant women are less at risk of physical abuse than younger women. Our own research does not contradict this, but this was mainly because very few women reported any sort of physical aggression:[9] when women were asked in a questionnaire whether arguments between themselves and their partner had ever come close to blows, the vast majority of women in both age groups (87 per cent) said 'never'.

During pregnancy women are routinely encouraged to adopt healthy lifestyles by not smoking or consuming alcohol, avoiding a high caffeine intake and certain 'high risk' foods, eating a nutritionally balanced diet, getting enough rest and exercise and so on. These issues are mentioned in Chapters 4 and 6 but here we shall return to them briefly in order to emphasize the way that family members are involved in improving or decreasing the chances that a woman will act in a way that gives her baby the best chances possible.

A study by one of the authors and colleagues suggests that giving up alcohol will depend on whether or not a woman feels she has adequate support, not just so far as abstaining from alcohol is concerned but in other areas of her life as well.[42] Furthermore, it is not just the helpful *intentions* of those around her that count, it is their *actions*. It is known that pregnant women with substance-abusing partners are nearly five times as likely to be substance-users themselves, compared with those who do not report that their partners use drugs.[43] One study of 529 women (aged 18–41) showed that women who lived with people who smoked, drank alcohol and/or caffeinated beverages were likely to smoke more or drink more themselves, (even if they felt that their partners were supportive of their intentions to abstain), compared with women trying to give up who lived with non-smokers/non-drinkers.[44] No comparison was made between older and younger mothers but the authors suggested that it might be important for health professionals to consider the families of pregnant women as well as the women themselves.

There are other examples of a mother's partnerships making a difference to her baby's well-being. For instance, it has been found that partner support can give rise to different effects depending on the women receiving the support: for white women, *lower levels* of partner support were associated with pre-term delivery, whereas for black women pre-term delivery was associated with *higher levels* of partner support.[45] Regardless of the explanation chosen for these findings, they clearly illustrate the complexity of the issue. Certainly, ethnic or cultural identity are important when trying to understand the effects of psychosocial environments on pregnancy and birth.[46]

Turning to the issue of psychological health, some researchers have found that even in the 1990s life is easier for married than unmarried couples, mainly because the former meet with higher levels of social approval and thus do not need to waste valuable energy defending their lifestyle.[47] They found that where partners were married, the members of the family related to each other more positively than was the case where partners lived together but were not married. They also found that family dynamics were more positive where maternal age was higher. The main message from studies of psychological well-being in families is that maternal age, *on its own*, tends not be be crucial: other things (social status, educational level, income etc.) are important too.

A study looking at marital satisfaction and the ways in which couples tried to cope with day-to-day situations found that when faced with a problem, married couples aged 20–29 were most likely out of all age groups to resort to conflict (sarcasm, criticism, revenge) and self-blame (worry, health or sleep problems, troubled feelings), but older couples used these negative strategies less and less often.[48] Thus women in the 35-plus group are less likely than younger women to engage in conflict or self-blame. At the same time, coping with problems by using gestures of physical affection and humour is something that increases after the age of 40.

∾

Looking ahead to the new family

One of the few studies that follows families until the child is three years old reported that families where parents were older had more education, a longer relationship and a higher income were more likely to say that the quality of their marriage improved over the time span of the study.[49] In a recent review Joan Aldous says that many researchers find that the presence of children in a marriage leads to reduced levels of marital satisfaction because partners do not get the chance to talk to each other as often as formerly, and because of an increase in financial problems.[50] However, there are those who argue that this reduction in companionship tends to happen over time, especially in the early years of marriage, whether or not a couple have children.[51]

Joan Aldous also points out that many researchers found that once a couple have a child the division of labour within the household becomes more 'traditional'. This tends to have a positive effect on the male partner (he likes it!) but a negative effect on the woman. It could pose particular problems for older first-time mothers as there is evidence to suggest that the longer women live apart from their parental families before establishing families of their own, the more likely they are to hold non-traditional gender role attitudes. A second potential pitfall here is that once members of a couple see themselves as unequal, which some people might argue could be one result of adopting traditional gender roles, they are less likely to confide in each other. However, rather than giving cause for concern these research findings may just reflect the various practical ways couples find of adapting to the demands of a new baby, and in any case older mothers tend to adopt less traditional gender roles than younger mothers, after birth.[10]

The nature of a couple's relationship is important not only because of its short-term effects but because of the way it affects family life in the long-term. In one long-term study it was found that women who felt that they and their partner were in agreement during pregnancy tended to say they were happier and felt more attached to the baby.[52] Furthermore they had a better quality of relationship with their children two years later. According to a long-term study by Jerry Lewis in the US, women's levels of anxiety and depression after birth can be predicted from the quality of the marriage before the birth: the better it is, the less likely it is that anxiety and depression will occur.[53] Any emotional turmoil following birth has usually passed by the time the baby reaches 12 months old, but recovery is quicker in women who were and are satisfied in their marriages.

In the long-term, so far as incorporating the child into the family is concerned, it has been found that it is the overall pattern of the marital relationship that matters. Different ways of coping (traditional gender roles, reversal of roles etc.) suit different people at different times in their marriage. In other words research has not found that there is any one type of 'ideal' marriage.

What are the implications of all the research, so far as older women and their new families are concerned? Chapter 10 takes further the discussion of family life after birth. For now suffice it to say that there is some evidence that the older the parents, the better the quality of their relationship with their child, the greater their satisfaction with being parents, and the higher their levels of well-being.[54]

↜ 8 ↝

Birth and Afterwards:
Facts and Feelings

It was just an experience really . . . when she was born I kept stroking her . . . she was perfect, not messy, no gunge – I saw other babies afterwards, with all matted hair. She was clean I couldn't believe it. I can't understand why people take videos, I can remember it (so clearly).
                                                  Dawn, 43 at birth of first baby

I was a bit 'out of it' not thinking about what I should do. My mind was whizzing round trying to concentrate on where my legs were and my head – I'd even forgotten I was having a baby, I was that confused at what was going on. I just burst into tears when I heard the cry. It was marvellous.
                                                  Karen, 36 at third birth

Many women comment on a curious phenomenon after they have had a baby. They describe how, when they are pregnant and look ahead into the future, they see only as far as giving birth and no further. 'Birth', at this point, means 'the end of pregnancy'. Then, once the baby is born, they find their perspective shifts dramatically and that they now see birth as a beginning – the beginning of the rest of their lives as a mother to the new arrival.

Many women have said after giving birth that they wished someone had prepared them beforehand for what their new life would be like; as Beryl pointed out at the end of Chapter 6 it is quite possible that becoming a mother is something that has to be experienced before it can be understood and that therefore even if information is provided during pregnancy about the postnatal period and the birth, it may not be fully comprehended until afterwards.

Birth can be seen as a sort of gateway, both the end of pregnancy and the beginning of a new life, rather like the Roman deity who is portrayed as looking in two directions at once to represent endings and beginnings simultaneously. How do older women experience their passage through this gateway?

Most research points to the fact that being older, on its own, is not particularly likely to influence the way labour and delivery progress and how women feel about it, except possibly for an increased risk of having a Caesarean section. Other factors such as a woman's health and whether or not she has given birth before tend to make more difference than maternal age alone. There is, therefore, no call for this chapter to attempt to replace the information given in many good manuals on childbirth which are useful to women of all ages.

The medical risks

In Chapter 5 we saw that older women who give birth in the 1990s are at a definite advantage compared with older women giving birth even a few decades ago, because they are likely to be a different type of woman: healthier, fewer previous pregnancies, more financially secure and so on. In addition they are likely to have been better monitored during pregnancy and any chronic conditions from which they suffer (for instance, diabetes or high blood pressure) are likely to be better controlled because of advances in medical understanding and management. Thus the outlook appears vastly better now than in the past for women giving birth at 35-plus. This contrast is even sharper when comparisons are made with conditions for older women two centuries ago, when 37 per cent of all first births occured to mothers over 35 according to one source.[1] These women were likely to have pelvic deformities, arising because they suffered from rickets as children, which could make delivery extremely difficult or impossible, as well as other chronic health problems such as respiratory TB. Figures from the 1880s suggest that 35-plus women expecting their first baby were then three times as likely to have forceps deliveries as younger first-timers.[1]

It was argued in Chapter 5 that 35-plus women may be at a slightly increased risk of developing pre-eclampsia (swelling, high blood pressure and protein in the urine), although this is not conclusively proven as being due to age alone and *may* not apply to white, middle-class, highly educated women. So far as placental complications are concerned, the more recent studies in which older mothers are typically having their first or second child suggest that women of 35-plus are not at an increased risk of complications. Older women who have given birth many times already *are* at a greater risk of placental complications.

The evidence concerning the relationship between a mother's age and how long her labour lasts is inconclusive because length of labour can be altered by the use of pain relief (more pain relief and longer labours go together) which in turn may depend partly on how concerned a mother and/or her birth attendants are about the mother's age. Overall there is no reason to assume that just because a woman is over 35 she will have a longer labour, although this has not always been the case: as recently as the 1960s, although only four per cent of women in general had labours lasting more than 24 hours, almost one quarter of first-time mothers over 35 had labours this long.[1] Today very few women are allowed to remain so long in labour.

Rates of Caesarean section have been found to be consistently higher for older women and this is only partly due to increased complications. It may reflect concern on the part of older mothers themselves and/or those who care for them. Thus at least some older mothers are more likely than younger women to have a Caesarean section, so we have included later in this chapter brief descriptions of women's feelings about the operation.

So far as the new baby is concerned, we concluded in Chapter 5 that being older does not mean that it is likely that the baby will be born 'pre-term'; although it is possible that older women may more often have very big, or low birthweight, babies. Findings about the health of the babies of older women are conflicting.

Some research seems to show that older women's babies are at risk of being less healthy at birth, other research does not. It seems that other things (number of previous children, mother's health and lifestyle etc.) may be more important than age alone. Infant death during or after birth is now very rare. Mothers over 35 are no more likely than younger women to lose their baby at or after birth, according to the studies we reviewed in Chapter 5.

꒰ꑇ

Do older women gain more weight during pregnancy?

By the end of pregnancy women may be somewhat concerned about the way they look and how their bodies feel. As Kathleen, aged 35, said when expecting her first baby: '*I felt listless and frumpy, uncomfy . . .*' and Wendy, whose weight went up from 73 to 91 kg (11 st 7 lbs to 14 st 5 lbs) was very concerned about this:

> *I've always had a weight problem – it's inherited. I started off lighter than with my first child and still ended up the same end weight. My GP was on at me all the time, constantly reminding me about too much weight gain . . .*
>
> *Age 36 at birth of second child*

In contrast, Fay, who was expecting her third baby, conceived by accident at 35, said: '*At one point I got told off for not putting any weight on.*'

There is some evidence that this sort of issue bothers younger women more than older women at late pregnancy.[2] Does age make a real difference to the amount of weight gained during pregnancy? One researcher says that older women are likely to gain more than younger women.[3] However, this may depend on other factors than age, such as level of education or occupation. In the Leicester Motherhood Project, where the older and younger groups had the same levels of education and occupation, it was found that among first-time mothers, older women put on significantly less weight than those in their twenties:[2] the average (i.e. mean) weight gain for 35-plus first-timers was 13.5 kg (2 st 1 lb) whereas the average weight gain for first-timers in their twenties was 18 kg (2 st 12 lbs). Women who had given birth before put on the same amount of weight (around 13.6 kg or 2 st 2 lbs) regardless of whether they were in their twenties or 35-plus.

๛

Preparation for labour: antenatal classes

Most women, regardless of age, feel at least a little anxious about the approaching labour. For instance, one study found that among first-time mothers, 73 per cent of older (35-plus) women and 71 per cent of younger (twenties) women were more than 'a bit' worried about the pain of labour.[2] This may be particularly true for those who have experienced any complications during late pregnancy.[4] How do women of 35-plus attempt to prepare themselves, emotionally and physically, for the event?

For 35-plus women who have already given birth before and have young children or other dependants, or for those who are in paid work, it may be difficult to attend birth preparation classes. Does this mean that older and younger women may differ in their levels of 'formal' preparation for labour?

Research by Lyn Quine and her colleagues suggests that older women are very likely to be better informed than younger women at late pregnancy.[5] However, she also points out that in the women she was comparing, more of the older ones were 'middle-class' – had non-manual occupations – and the younger ones were largely working-class, more of them having manual occupations. The working-class women found the classes less useful because they preferred not to discuss their questions and concerns in front of the middle-class women, whereas the middle-class women had no such inhibitions, presumably partly because the teachers were also perceived as middle-class. However, one researcher argues that working-class women benefit more from classes than do middle-class women.[6]

There is some evidence that attending classes can help new mothers to feel that they have some control over what happens during labour.[7] A recent report by Dutch researchers reviews much of the evidence on the effects of attending classes.[8] Overall, they say studies suggest that attending childbirth preparation classes cannot influence how long labour will be or the incidence of complications, and this is supported by the findings of an Austrian study.[9] However, there are some benefits. One group of researchers found that first-time mothers, asked about classes after they had given birth, said that antenatal classes were more helpful than they had expected them to be.[10] American reviewers argue, unlike the Dutch report, that those who attend classes may have fewer physical complications during labour, and improved physical health after the birth.[11] Higher levels of preparation tend to go with lower use of pain relief during labour.[8] However, this review points out that authors express concern about childbirth preparation classes in case they lead to unrealistic expectations about labour pain and hence disappointment, because as one researcher put it: 'Labour is still painful after childbirth training.'[12]

꒰

The experience of labour after 35

Overall, the research evidence from several countries including the UK, Sweden, Austria, Netherlands and the US tends to suggest that there are relatively few differences between younger and older women in the way they experience labour.[8, 9, 13, 14, 15] This tallies with the relative similarity in medical expectations for older and younger women today – barring Caesarean section – so long as age is not confounded by other factors such as chronic ill-health or parity (the number of previous children born to a woman). Three themes emerge when reading the literature on women's subjective experiences of labour. These are concerned with women's *expectations* about what labour and delivery will be like, *the level of control* a woman feels she has over what is happening – whether or not she feels as if things are just 'being done to her' without permission or whether her relationship with the staff is more equable – and with the importance of having some sort of *emotional support* during labour.

Expectations and reality

These days many women, perhaps particularly those expecting their first baby after 35, have high expectations for their experience of labour. They do not have much chance to 'practise' giving birth as they are likely to have only one or two children, so they may feel that they want to 'get it right' first time. Does having high expectations sow the seed for eventual disappointment?

Very few studies have looked at the way age might or might not influence women's expectations about labour. Results of the Leicester Motherhood Project suggest that older first-time mothers *may* have higher expectations of personal fulfilment during labour than younger women.[2] Among first-time 35-plus mothers, 70 per cent said that they hoped that labour and delivery would definitely be a 'really fulfilling experience' for them, compared with 54 per cent of those in their twenties. The corresponding figures for experienced mothers were 50 and 57 per cent for 35-plus and 20–29 year-olds respectively. In another study age was not related to childbirth expectations although there is other evidence that older women, and more educated women, may have generally higher expectations of themselves, which might explain the Leicester Motherhood Project findings.[4, 16]

Most women giving birth after 35 have done so before; might their previous experience influence their expectations? Gerd Fridh and Fannie Gaston-Johannson found that the answer is probably 'no'.[17] Both first-time and experienced mothers in their study underestimated the amount of pain and discomfort they would undergo during labour. However, women who had already given birth before were pleasantly surprised to find that they did not need so much medication as they had anticipated, and that they had better self-control than they had expected. Those who expected labour to be more painful found that it actually was more painful. Was this because they were good at assessing their own pain thresholds – or could it be that 'if you expect the worst you get the worst'?

Are 'great expectations' a bad thing?

Josephine Green and her co-workers in Cambridge, UK, are interested in this issue. In their study of 825 women they found that having high expectations about labour was *not* bad for women: but expecting the worst could sometimes be followed by bad experiences.[18] They said that most women found birth fulfilling, and those who expected it to be fulfilling were more likely to find that it had been so. Those who expected it to be painful were likely to find that it was, but on the positive side, those who wanted to try to cope without drugs were more likely to do so and were more satisfied with the birth experience, and those who expected to find breathing and relaxation to be useful were more likely to find that this was so. Furthermore, if women expected to feel in control of themselves and what happened to them they were likely to achieve this aim and to feel happy and contented (not depressed) after the birth.

The important message from this research is that women with high expectations of themselves and birth are *not* bound to be disappointed and dissatisfied. Anne Byrne-Lynch in Ireland agrees that having a general belief in one's ability to cope with labour is a 'powerful positive influence on subsequent performance in this situation'.[19] She also makes the point that high expectations, or belief in ability to cope, are not to be confused with:

An unthinking optimism which foolishly ignores the possible negative aspects of the forthcoming childbirth experience. It is rather a belief that most women have some personal resources which they can mobilise to meet what will be a very personally challenging situation.

How do older women feel about being in control during labour?

There are obviously many aspects of a labour and delivery that lie outside anyone's control, but nevertheless women still appreciate not finding themselves in a situation where they feel '*like a slab of meat*', as one woman put it. One such unfortunate experience is described by Wendy:

> *I had an internal* [vaginal examination] *and the midwife said 'your waters are bulging – and I'm not coming in here again* [i.e. giving another vaginal examination] *because of infection risk, so do you want me to break them or not?' Under pressure I said yes . . . I lost control after the waters were broken and again when they were putting in the epidural. It was just so uncomfortable. For one contraction I lost my breathing and the midwife said 'come on . . . this is labour. It's hard work, that's why it's called labour.' I thought 'You wait till your turn.'*
>
> *Age 36 at birth of second child*

The majority of women of 35-plus did not recount such negative feelings. As Kathleen said:

> *You think you're losing control but actually your body takes over . . . you're still doing the breathing but you feel slightly detached – the pain goes, the gas and air are still there – you feel as if you're someone else but then another pain comes and [I] realize it's me.*
>
> *Age 35 at birth of first child*

and Lesley, when asked about whether she had felt in control of what the staff were doing to her, said: 'there was nobody in control except my body'. Stephanie had a slightly different view-point, but nevertheless felt happy that control was not being taken away from her:

> *It was what the baby was doing that was the controlling factor, rather than the staff or me.*
>
> *Age 35 at birth of first child*

173

Given that 'feeling in control' is important, is there any evidence that older women are more likely to feel in control during labour? Josephine Green did not report any association with maternal age, and also said that level of education did not make a difference to the extent to which feeling in control was important.[18] In the Leicester Motherhood Project, whose findings may be particularly relevant for women in non-manual occupations with a fairly high level of education, it was found that age made no difference to women's feelings about their relationship with the staff so far as control was concerned. Regardless of age, 76 per cent said they were happy, or mostly happy, with the way the staff treated them and 78 per cent were satisfied with the level of explanation they had received. When asked whether they felt in control of what the staff were doing to them, 61 per cent said 'all or most of the time' as compared with only 17 per cent who said 'hardly at all'. The majority of women did not feel that they had lost control of the way they themselves had behaved during labour. Looking only at first-time mothers, age appeared to be an advantage here because 62 per cent of 35-plus first-timers said they 'definitely never lost control', compared with only 44 per cent of first-time mothers in their twenties.

Pain in labour

Women who have given birth tend to agree that pain in labour is different from other sorts of pain. One difference is that it is intermittent – coming in waves. Furthermore it increases in severity as time goes by – each wave tends to be more severe than the waves before; but most importantly it is different because it is 'pain with a purpose' – each contraction brings the baby's arrival one step closer. It is sometimes easy to lose sight of this last feature, according to women's reports of labour.

There is no evidence to suggest that women of 35-plus need to worry that they will experience more pain in labour than younger women, although this may simply be because, as we pointed out earlier, the majority of women tend to underestimate the pain of labour. As Lesley said, when asked whether there was any point at which the pain was worse than she had expected it to be:

Yes, right at the beginning! I must have forgotten. If I'd remembered I'd never have had another. I don't like pain, I can't be noble about it.
Age 38 at birth of second child

And Heather:

I knocked the midwives across the floor and practically broke my husband's hand. Even now when I hear the word 'push' it jumps out at me – they said it a lot because he was distressed . . . They all said I was very brave because I didn't scream – but I had no puff, the pain was so bad . . . I find birth horrendous. There's nothing enjoyable about it, except the little bundle at the end.
Age 38 at birth of second child

There were many who painted a more positive picture, even of the pain. Jackie had given birth to a son three years previously and had had a very difficult labour lasting 22½ hours, during which she said she had 'everything' in the way of interventions and medication. However, her more recent delivery was an entirely positive experience. She had asked to be induced because of her previous experience and said:

Even the timing was excellent. I could choose to come in on Sunday and give birth on Monday. It was quite funny going in with a suitcase thinking 'I'll come out with a baby.'
Age 40 at birth of second child

She used only gas and air, and the only point at which she said the pain had been worse than she had anticipated 'to some extent' was just before the baby was born and this was

Only because it took so long last time [that] *I thought I might be in for another 10 hours . . . The staff were wonderful – they asked whether I'd like her on my stomach . . . I said I couldn't care less!* [Husband] *held her and I took the picture* [when she was born], *I had no desperate need to hold her . . . I had a male midwife and a student who made a point of seeing me after the birth on the ward, and of carrying the baby out for me when she heard we were going.*

Pain relief for older mothers

There was a tendency among participants in the Leicester Motherhood Project for older first-time mothers to be slightly less happy with the pain relief they used, compared with younger first-timers.[2] They were less likely to use pethidine than younger women, but the numbers receiving general anaesthesia, or using 'gas and air', epidural or spinal blocks did not vary with age. Another study found that older women were less likely than younger women to choose epidural anaesthesia.[21] In this study, the older women tended to be active rather than passive participants in labour, and were likely to feel that control over the situation did not rest solely with the medical professionals. Anne Byrne-Lynch found some evidence that women who opt for epidurals, looking back on delivery, are likely to feel that they had levels of pain that were lower than those remembered by women using pethidine or no pain relief.[20] However, pain levels reported by those using pethidine were just as high as those experienced by those using no pain relief. In other words, at least for some women, pethidine does not necessarily relieve pain although it may have effects which make the pain more tolerable. Epidural anaesthesia does relieve pain but has been found to go hand in hand with feeling less 'in control'. This does not mean that opting for epidural anaesthesia *necessarily* leads to losing control: it may be that women opt for an epidural partly *because* they prefer to leave the progress of labour in the hands of the professionals.

At what point in labour do women opt for pain relief, and why? Is it when they reach a certain intensity of pain? Some research suggests that this is not so, because women who choose pain relief do not necessarily feel more pain, just before opting for medication, than the level experienced by those who did not have medication.[20] Possibly the length of time for which pain has to be endured is important here. What are also important are women's feelings about whether or not they are going to be able to cope. Anne Byrne-Lynch found that it was possible to predict at late pregnancy which women would use pain relief in labour: those who were least confident in their coping ability were most likely to use pain relief.[20] Pain relief during labour is very much a matter of personal choice with different options suiting different women at different points in labour. As Winne said when asked what advice she would pass on to other women of 35-plus:

> *Keep an open mind about pain relief . . . in delivery – be prepared for things not to go as planned in your ideal situation – apart from an epidural I intended to have anything I could – in the event I had nothing! It's all well worth the effort. Rocking from side to side whilst standing does appear to release your natural painkillers. Gravity (I believe) is one of the most helpful ways to speed up labour – deliver as vertically as possible.*
>
> *Age 40 at birth of second child*

Women's satisfaction with the experience of giving birth, when they look back on the experience, does not always depend on the level of pain relief. In one study, for instance, those who were *least* satisfied about the way things had gone were those who had had the *most effective* pain relief.[20] In the Leicester Motherhood Project, both older and younger women felt that they coped well with the pain – 83 per cent said they coped 'quite well' or 'very well'.

Do older women perceive intervention differently?

One finding from the Leicester Motherhood Project was particularly interesting. Although age made no difference to the extent to which women felt in control of themselves or of the staff, it did seem to affect the chances that staff were perceived as doing things that made labour pains worse such as requiring them to adopt a position that was uncomfortable.

For example, one of only four older, first-time mothers who had this experience said:

I was not happy with the last hour altogether, because until then I'd been taken through it by the midwife. Then there was a change of shift and the new midwife had me on all fours – I hated it, I felt like a dog. She wouldn't let me move, said it was the best position for the baby. But I couldn't push like that, I wanted to be on my side.

Helena, 35 at birth of first baby

However, overall older women did *not* feel this strongly. This age difference was particularly true for first-time mothers, such that 63 per cent of women in their twenties said that someone else had done something that made the pain worse, as opposed to only 16 per cent of 35-plus first-time mothers.

It is difficult to explain this age difference in terms of obstetric interventions or other events because younger first-timers were not more likely than older women to have interventions which might be painful. (Things that did not happen more frequently among younger mothers were induction, augmention, artificial rupture of membranes, Caesarean section, delivery via forceps or ventouse, episiotomy, tearing or stitching: rates tended to be the same among first-timers regardless of age). Thus the explanation may lie in differing perceptions or interpretations of other people's actions by older and younger women, and this in turn may depend on the relative ages of the women themselves and those who were caring for them. In this study data on the midwives' and obstetricians' ages, relative to the ages of the women they attended, were not collected so this hypothesis could not be tested. There is room for further research here. Certainly, older women's perceptions of the midwives attending them tended to be positive, as Tina described:

The last midwife was very nice, very encouraging. She used my name, and she got it right . . . she sat on the bed and rubbed my back.

Age 39 at birth of third child

Among first-time mothers, older and younger women's percep-tions of the way staff handled things differed in another situation – that which arose when there had been some suggestion that the baby might be having problems. Older women's babies were no more likely to have problems than were younger women's, according to the mothers' own accounts, but more older than younger women said that they were definitely happy with the way this situation was handled (83 per cent versus 53 per cent). Somewhat paradoxically, younger women (44 per cent of them) were more likely than older women (23 per cent) to say that it had 'never crossed their mind' that the baby's life might be in danger.

Emotional support during labour

We have already pointed out the importance, regardless of age, of not feeling as if things are 'being done to you without permission' during labour. Another factor that emerges as important in assessments of women's experiences of labour is that of feeling psychologically supported by a companion.

Findings relating support during labour to maternal age are scarce, although some researchers do touch on age. For instance, Lyn Quine found that older women (who were also of higher socio-economic status) tended to be better supported than younger women at late pregnancy and that high levels of support tended to go hand in hand with feeling less pain during labour.[5]

The importance of at least one companion during labour itself has been recognized throughout history in a wide range of cultures, as Monique Bydlowski points out, although it is only relatively recently, according to her and other sources that men, including the baby's father, have been involved in birth.[22, 1] Dwenda Gjerdingen and her colleagues, in their review of many recent studies on support, found that mothers who had the support of a companion during labour and delivery experienced fewer childbirth complications and less depression after the birth.[11] The therapeutic effects of a companion still operate even if the companion is only a silent observer.[23]

Caesarean section

In Chapter 5 we said that the only intervention that is more likely to be experienced by older than younger women is Caesarean section, although in the Leicester Motherhood Project it was found that this difference did not appear.[2] In that study, analysis included only those women who had agreed to take part in a long-term study (around half of those initially approached), so the women are not typical of the general population. In addition, recruitment focused on a single hospital, and it is, of course, possible that hospitals vary in the extent to which factors other than the purely obstetric influence their decisions about operative deliveries. However, the findings are nevertheless of value because levels of occupation and education were the same for older and younger groups of first-time and 'experienced' mothers and there may in some cases be a link between educational qualifications or occupation, and obstetric intervention. For instance, Sandra Elliott and others in a British study found that women with more educational qualifications were less likely to be induced, and speculated as to whether this meant that less educated women had more complications or that highly educated women put up more resistance to induction.[13]

Women who know in advance that they will be having a Caesarean section may be likely to be well-prepared for the operation, as Michelle said:

> *I was pleased to have a Caesar, especially as I have problems with piles and varicose veins – I'd been on the sick for months, it was not an easy pregnancy . . . There were ten people there* [in the operating room] *laughing and joking . . . it was a really different atmosphere from when you're stuck in labour. I really enjoyed it – it was luxury compared with labour, and I was very well looked after.*
>
> Age 37 at birth of third child

However, for those who find the need for a Caesarean section arises as an emergency once they have already gone into labour, the shock can be considerable regardless of age.

I had not prepared to have a Caesarean as I had two natural births and still feel baffled about it and still do not know exactly what they did to me during the operation. I think Caesarean birth should be discussed in detail at parentcraft classes or antenatal visits.

Karen, age 36 at birth of third child
after a long gap following divorce and remarriage

Karen still felt very strongly that she didn't know what had happened to her when she was interviewed a year after the birth. Jenny, in her twenties, echoes these feelings:

I wish someone had told me more of the details about a Caesarean birth – although it was mentioned at antenatal [classes], *it was not explained thoroughly. The midwife running the class said, when asked about Caesareans, 'well, you won't be needing one, will you?'*

In the event Jenny had a failed forceps delivery and had to be delivered by Caesarean section.

Given that older women as a group are more likely to undergo Caesarean section it would seem sensible to recommend that information about what happens during a Caesarean is made available to those older women who wish for it. As pointed out in Chapter 6, information about a medical condition or procedure can be helpful in allaying anxiety, and is most unlikely to have a negative effect.

CAESAREAN SECTION:
WHAT HAPPENS IN THE OPERATION (BOX 8.1)

Anaesthesia
A woman may have epidural anaesthesia, which means that she can remain conscious during the operation, or she may have a general anaesthetic. The operation will not be started until surgeons have checked that the anaesthetic has worked. With epidural anaesthesia the mother cannot see the operation but she can hear the baby's first cry and can hold the baby as soon as a quick medical check has been made. The baby's father may be more likely to be allowed to watch the delivery if epidural anaesthesia is used, and there is evidence that his presence has positive effects:[24] He can

cont.

---

support the mother and help convey her feelings to the medical staff, apart from the benefits of being involved in such a momentous occasion as the birth of their child.

The incisions and delivery
The incision may be *vertical* (up and down in the mid-line below the navel) or *transverse* (side-to-side across the lower abdomen) so that once it has healed it will be covered up by the pubic hair (which is shaved for the operation). There is a layer of muscles under the surface which is separated to reach the abdominal cavity, at which point the surgeon can see the bladder and other internal organs. The bladder is carefully freed from the lower part of the womb, so that the surgeon can make an incision from side-to-side through the wall of the womb. Then she or he can see the membranes surrounding the baby, which are also parted, and the baby's head is delivered. Before delivering the body the baby's face will be wiped and mucus cleared from her or his mouth and nose. After the body is delivered the umbilical cord is clamped as usual, and the baby would probably be given first to a midwife who is in the room.

The placenta
From the parents' and baby's point of view the most important part of the operation is now over: it usually takes only about 10 minutes. However, the mother cannot be stitched up until the womb contracts, which it does about 40 seconds after an injection of ergometrine or syntometrine, and until the placenta has been delivered through the same incision as the baby.

Repairing the incisions
Stitching now begins. Once the womb has contracted it is stitched using either two or three layers of stitches. The Fallopian tubes and ovaries are checked, and if everything is normal the muscular wall of the abdomen is stitched in four layers, using different stitches for different layers. The skin incision is then closed either with stitches or with clips.

The information given here is taken from Gordon Bourne's book, *Pregnancy*.[25]

⤳

The new baby

No description of labour and delivery would be complete without some mention of the baby. Research has not looked in detail at differences between 35-plus and younger women in the ways they respond to their new baby. As has been apparent throughout this chapter, age alone does not appear to be particularly important here, at birth, although there may be slight differences between older and younger women's feelings in the months and years that follow. For instance, women of 35-plus may say that they can tell 'what sort of a person' their baby is earlier than younger women. Similarly they are likely to say their baby 'became a sociable person' earlier than mothers in their twenties, and this is not due to any difference in biological age (i.e. since conception). In Chapter 10 we delve further into this under-researched area and look at whether a 35-year (or more) generation gap makes a difference.

Returning to birth, Jenny's reflections on things she found help-ful after a difficult delivery are likely to ring true regardless of age:

The comment which helped me most was not to expect too much too soon – i.e. that I would not necessarily feel immediate love for my child. After a difficult birth, I didn't and was relieved when I remembered this was not either unusual or wrong. Time is very important. It heals and enables life to return to a certain degree of normality!
Jenny, age 25 at birth of first child

Older women's reactions to their babies are as varied as those of any other age group.

I said hello. I noticed how weird he looked – the texture of his skin – it was blue . . . he was like a being from outer space.
Marta, age 35 at birth of second child by Caesarean section

It was like greeting someone different from what you'd expected. He looked familiar and unfamiliar.
Fay, age 35 at birth of third child

183

I didn't expect him to look so small or so badly bruised.
Janice, age 36, baby born at 28 weeks' gestation. This baby recovered completely from his premature delivery and was a healthy, sociable little boy when we interviewed her one year after the birth.

I was just staring at her and being absolutely amazed and delighted. It was wonderful, wonderful . . .

Isabel, 35, first child – (see Chapter 2)

⁓

Physical recovery from childbirth

Is it harder for older women to 'get back to normal' after giving birth? When asked whether she had done so, three months after birth, Lesley said:

I don't know, because I've got to find my new 'normal'. I don't think I'll ever be normal . . . I feel a wreck, physically, I can't find time to get my hair cut – you see chic women and you're covered in marmite or milk.

Age 38 at birth of second child

Experiences vary in this respect: Margaret had her fourth child at 35 and said she was completely back to normal ten weeks after the birth, apart from feeling more tired than previously. Expectations also vary: Valerie, having her second child at 41, said:

I was a little concerned [about getting back to normal] *– with my first child I could get back into my* [pre-pregnancy] *dress within a week. This time it shocked me – I couldn't carry a basket of washing to the back door at eight days* [after delivery] *. . . it took longer than I thought. I'm still not at full strength* [at four months].

In one study of women six months after childbirth, 25 per cent did not feel fully recovered by this time, particularly if they had had a long labour or a Caesarean section.[26] One reviewer estimates that as many as one third of women delivered by Caesarean section have an infection afterwards.[27] Older women may be likely to stay in hospital longer than younger women and to describe hospital routines as stressful.[14]

In the British study of 40-plus mothers it was found that women giving birth for the first time over 40 said that it had taken around 11 months, on average, before they felt physically 'back to normal'.[28] Women of 40-plus who were not first-timers said it had taken seven to eight months on average. First-time and experienced mothers did not differ on the amount of 'bother' caused by any physical changes they had experienced in the first year, and for both groups the most frequently noted changes were in stomachs, breasts, bladder control and backs. In the Leicester Motherhood Project, it was found that more older than younger mothers said they had suffered from stress incontinence or extreme tiredness at some time during the first year after birth, but more younger than older women had had headaches during the first year.[2] These findings mirror those from a study of over 11,000 British women who gave birth between 1978 and 1985. In this study, too, more older than younger mothers reported bladder problems and fatigue during the first year after birth.[29] However, what stands out from the findings of this very large study is the *infrequency* with which being older was associated with having problems with health after childbirth. In fact, older women were sometimes at an advantage: for instance they seemed less likely to suffer from the type of headache that is associated with being under social stresses.

When women in the Leicester Motherhood Project were asked whether there had been anything for which they had not felt prepared, and would like to pass on to help other women, two commented on the lochia – the normal vaginal discharge after birth.[2] There is no standard duration of bleeding after delivery; in some women it stops after two weeks, in some it goes on for six weeks or so.[25] We have not found any suggestion that it lasts longer for older women, but include Alison's comment as reassurance that a long lochia can be normal:

I was not prepared for the yuckiness of lochia – a closely guarded secret and the last thing one feels in need of dealing with when one has a new baby, stitches etc. The first time it went on for six weeks – ugh.

Age 39 at birth of second child

Whether or not a woman breastfeeds her baby may affect how long it takes her to 'feel back to normal'. Some women find they have no problems with breastfeeding but others find it extremely difficult:

I had such problems because he had a small mouth . . . I was terribly sore – if it hadn't been for moral and physical support [from midwives and partner] I would've given up.

Marta, 35 at birth of second child

I got sore very quickly and I thought it could have been avoided. I never had the same midwife supervising me and I was never watched for a whole feed . . . The whole experience was as bad as labour . . . you couldn't see the end to it. My husband helped; he said try to keep going – because neither of us could stand the thought of bottles! . . . Mind you, it caused a lot of merriment too – we'd never seen an E cup [bra] before!

Ann, 37 at birth of first child

It has been suggested that women who feel depressed during pregnancy may have more physical difficulties with breast-feeding, but this does not mean that older women are at a disadvantage because they may suffer less from depression during pregnancy than younger women, as we suggested in Chapter 6.[30] Breastfeeding is discussed further in Chapter 10.

ᣩ

Emotional well-being after childbirth

In Chapter 6 we looked at the evidence showing that older women did not seem to be at a greater risk of depression during pregnancy than younger women, and in Chapter 7 we pointed out that emotional support was one important 'protector' against suffering from depression. Here, we shall look a little more closely at older mothers' emotions after childbirth.

Looking back four months after her first baby's birth, Kim said:

I was not prepared for how differently I would feel being a mother. A mother and wife first and then somewhere in the background, me as a person.

Age 35

Was she suffering from postnatal depression, or was her reaction typical enough to be seen as normal? On the basis of one quote alone it is impossible to say. What is postnatal depression, how can women tell whether they are suffering from it, and how common is it among women of 35-plus? The consensus is that it is convenient to divide emotional disturbances that can affect women after birth into three types, although there are researchers in the field who are careful to point out that in real life 'there are no natural dividing points for distinguishing between various subtypes of postpartum affective disorders.'[31]

One extreme type of 'postpartum affective disorder' (i.e. an emotional disturbance that can affect women after birth) is extremely rare, touching only two in every thousand women, and it is known as postpartum psychosis because its symptoms include auditory hallucinations (hearing things that are not there) and paranoid delusions (for instance, believing that others are conspiring against one).

One of the more usual, but in some ways less serious sorts of disturbance is something often described as 'the blues'. Ruth York has studied 'the blues' and says that between 50 and 80 per cent of women will experience the condition.[32] It is not strictly 'depression' in the sense of feeling sad or miserable, rather it is a state of being generally very emotional – perhaps easily moved to tears by either intense joy or intense despair – with moods changing from day to day. She says symptoms tend to rise to a peak between the third to seventh day after delivery, and that this may be related to length of stay in hospital, although the same pattern emerges in many different countries including Africa, the UK and the US, where hospital stays may not all be of the same length, if experienced at all. By the tenth to fourteenth day after delivery the number of women suffering symptoms decreases. (There is nothing magical about days seven, ten or fourteen, it is just that she used these days to ask women for information. So a woman who is still having symptoms on day 15 does not need to feel unduly concerned.) This type of emotional disturbance usually disappears without the need for formal treatment.

Jacqueline Thirkettle and Robert Knight reviewed relevant research and found no connection between raised maternal age and a woman's chances of suffering from the blues.[33] There is some evidence that what happens during childbirth may slightly relate to having the blues, particularly if birth was difficult and painful, and the mother was very anxious, felt dissatisfied with how she coped and so on.[34] Depression during a pregnancy that is otherwise trouble-free may make the blues more likely.

The other sort of emotional disturbance is usually described as 'postnatal depression'. This is experienced by between 10 and 50 per cent of women, depending partly on how different researchers have described and measured it, and also partly on the women who are taking part in the research. For instance a study which found rates as high as 50 per cent was carried out in Israel at the time of the war with Lebanon, a period when many husbands spent some time on army reserve duty which may have involved time at the front, so the higher incidence of depression may have been due to stresses associated with war.[35] Postnatal depression has been defined variously as 'as psychiatric complication of the postpartum period,'[36] or as:

> an association of prolonged dysphoric mood [i.e. feeling ill at ease], lack of interest in activities and the somatic symptoms of depression (e.g. sleep disturbances, anorexia, fatigue)[37]

More recent researchers point out that it is not sensible to regard symptoms such as recent weight change and fatigue as signs that women are depressed after birth, as these are a normal part of the postpartum period, so definitions of postnatal depression these days centre on its emotional and 'thinking' elements. For instance, symptoms mentioned in a scale currently used to help assess whether or not women are suffering from depression include lack of ability to 'see the funny side of things' or look forward to things, blaming oneself unnecessarily, feeling anxious or panicky without good reason, feeling sad, unhappy or as if things have been getting on top of one, crying, and thinking about harming oneself.[38] This sort of depression lasts longer than the blues, and may extend at least throughout the first year after delivery.[39] It also starts later than the blues, but many women who suffer from it are already depressed in pregnancy.[18, 35, 40]

There are some studies[41, 42] which suggest that older women are sometimes more at risk from postnatal depression than younger women, but in these studies the effects of age could be confounded by, for example, the fact that the older women may have had more Caesarean sections, and this could be what makes them depressed.[41-45] There is other evidence suggesting that older women are not at greater risk than younger women and may even be less likely to suffer from depression.[2, 46] Overall, studies regarding rates of postnatal depression among older women suggest that increased age alone is unlikely to lead to high rates of depression.[47, 48]

Emotional support after birth

Many studies (*see Chapter* 7) indicate that one important feature that separates depressed from non-depressed mothers is how well-supported they feel by friends and family.[27, 49] Whether or not older women have more emotional support was also discussed in Chapter 7. We mentioned the different sorts of support provided by friends (emotional support) and family (practical support), and said that in some situations families can be sources of stress rather than of help, although this is not always the case.

In studies which have looked at maternal age and the extent to which mothers have close ties with others, most, but not all, find that being older does not put women at a disadvantage and may put them at an advantage, depending on their cultural back-ground.[50] One study found that among African American mothers, age did influence how often women moved house – older ones moved less often – but in any case house-moves tended to be within one area so close ties were not disrupted.[51] Swedish mothers' ages did not influence how often they moved or how often close ties were disrupted. White American mothers, for whom kin support is usually very important, were less likely to rely on their families if they were highly educated. Older white American mothers were less likely than younger ones to have close ties disrupted.

Birth as a positive experience

Postnatal depression and a lack of support are not likely to be particular problems for older women. Although we have discussed them this should not obscure the fact that many researchers find that giving birth can give rise to very positive feelings. It has even been suggested that childbirth (although paradoxically, not pregnancy) can to some extent have a protec-tive effect against anxiety and depression.[52]

To sum up; there are many factors more important than a woman's age that affect how she feels about stepping across the threshold that birth represents. As Sandra Elliott, a psychologist and mother wrote:

> It seems to me that all the data confirm that which most parents know intuitively – that births change lives, that these changes are not necessarily predictable and that the changes are as vari-able as the pre-existing lives or indeed as variable as babies!

✌ 9 ✌

Multiple Roles, Multiple Lives: Making Decisions about Paid Work

Most women who have their first child at 35-plus and many of those who complete their families at this age will have spent more time in paid employment and invested more energy in career development than those who have children younger. This is true whether later motherhood is a result of choice or circumstance. Of course, this does not mean that women having children later are any less committed to motherhood. Indeed, many will have given lengthy consideration to the decision to have a child and others will have spent many years attempting to conceive. For a woman having a child later, decisions about whether to return to paid employment after the birth of the child are, therefore, particularly important. Are 35-plus mothers more likely to return to paid employment than younger mothers? If so, what choices do they make about the care of their child? These issues are the subject of the first part of this chapter.

Having a baby challenges previously held identity and priorities. After becoming a mother there is less time for paid work because of the new responsibilities and the practical constraints of day-care availability. A woman's view of herself and that of others, particularly of work colleagues and other mothers, will invariably change. How do women cope with their multiple roles? What is the impact of these on health, well-being and self identity? These issues are addressed in the second part of this chapter.

ぷ

Decisions about returning to paid work

The participation of women in the workforce in Western societies such as those of the US and Britain, has increased dramatically over the past two decades. This pattern has been particularly marked among women with children under school age.[1-4] In Britain, for example, between 1981 and 1991 the number of women with children under the age of five rose from 24 to 44 per cent.[4] Despite this rapid change, women with young children who do paid work remain a minority. We have not yet reached a point where most mothers of pre-school children are in paid employment (*see Table 9.1*). Moreover, very few are in full-time employment. Julia Brannen and Peter Moss point out that only a handful of women remain in the labour force throughout their child-bearing and child-rearing years and less than one in five return to paid work within the first nine months of their child's life.[3] A typical pattern is for a woman to work intermittently throughout the early years of motherhood with a mixture of part-time work and time away from full-employment.[2]

These patterns reflect the difficult decisions women have to make about paid employment once they are mothers. The family's financial needs and the desire to maintain career are placed up against concerns about care for the child and the adequacy of non-maternal child care. There are also social pressures which dictate that 'a mother's place is in the home'.[5]

Are 35-plus mothers more likely to return to paid work?

Women who have become mothers at a whole range of ages and at different stages in their careers can be found in the workforce. What distinguishes those who have their children later? Perhaps the single most evident characteristic of women who have their children later are that they are more likely to have a higher level of educational qualification and be in higher status occupations than those who time their children earlier.[6-8] Though extended periods of education necessitate delayed entrance into the workforce, there is evidence that women who time their children later have spent more time in paid work before having children. In the Australian Timing of Motherhood study three quarters of the women had worked for at least ten years prior to having children compared with less than half of average timing mothers (25–29 years) and none of the early timing mothers (less than 24 years) (*see Table 9.2*). These figures suggest that women who have their children later have a greater investment in career.

Table 9.1. Proportion of women with pre-school children who are in paid employment in selected countries

Country	Not seeking work %	Unemployed %	Employed %
United Kingdom (1985)	61	11	29
USA (1986)	46	6	48
Australia (1986)	59	4	37
Germany (1985)	61	7	32
France (1985)	41	9	50
Denmark (1995)	16	12	73

Source: Brannen & Moss, 1988[1]

Studies of women working in a range of higher status occupations provide evidence that they are more likely to return to work after having a child. In different occupations the ease of combining career and motherhood varies and the way in which this is managed varies, however. For those working in the business world, the environment seems to be most hostile to motherhood.

Women in management are less likely to have children than those in other occupations and those that do are faced with an 'all or nothing' situation. They feel pressured to minimize the amount of interference to their career by limiting the amount of leave they take for child-bearing and by returning on a full-time basis.[9, 10] There is evidence that women working in this sphere limit their family size.[11] Women working in other professional spheres appear to be more able to negotiate a range of options including combinations of part-time work and flexible hours and leave arrangements to combine work with motherhood. The findings that women in higher status occupations are more likely to return to paid work and that women having children after 35 are more likely to have a higher occupation together suggest that late timing mothers are more likely to return to work.

Table 9.2. Number of years worked prior to having children for early (less than 25 years), average (25–29 years) and late timing mothers (30 years and over)

Years worked	Early %	Average %	Late %
None	18	0	0
1–5	48	7	2
6–10	34	47	23
10 or more	0	47	75

Source: Thorpe & Cinnamon, Australian Timing of Motherhood study[6]

Is there any direct evidence of the relationship between timing of motherhood and return to the workforce? There is surprisingly little information on this subject. Two studies report on return to work after the birth of a first child only. In the Australian Timing of Motherhood Study women were asked if they had returned to work after the birth of their first child. In a comparison of early (under 25), average (between 25 and 29) and late (30 or more) mothers a higher proportion of those in the average and late timing group returned to work but this was not statistically significant. When the late timing group was divided into those between 30 and 34 and those aged 35 or more, greater differences were evident. Among 35-plus mothers those who did not work were a small minority; 18 per cent, compared with 27 per cent of mothers aged 30 to 34 and 36 per cent of those aged 20 to 25 at the time of their first birth (*see Table 9.3*). A study from the US also found that women who had their first child after the age of 35 were more likely to return to work.[12] This study compared a group of women having their first child over the age of 35 and a group aged 31 or less at their first birth. Twelve months after the birth of their first child all the women in the late timing group had returned to work compared with only a third of the younger timing group. The British study of 40-plus mothers, however, which included both women having their first and those having a subsequent child, found that less than half (45 per cent) returned to work after having their child.[13]

Table 9.3. Percentage of women returning to work according to timing of first birth

Timing of first birth	Returned %	Did not return %
Early timing (under 25 years)	32	64
Average timing (25–29 years)	73	27
Late timing (30 or more years)	73	27
30–34 years	73	27
35+	82	18

Source: Thorpe & Cinnamon, Australian Timing of Motherhood study[6]

The information on the hours worked by mothers according to the age at which they became mothers is very limited. In the US study the only information provided is that some of the women had returned to work on a part-time basis.[12] The Australian Timing of Motherhood study provides more detail.[6] In this study there were no differences in the number of hours worked per week by early, average and late timing mothers. Within each group the amount of time in paid work ranged from a few hours to over 40 hours per week.

Reasons for returning to paid work

Why do women work after they have become mothers? Are the motivations to do paid work different for late timing mothers than for other groups? For women with young children paid work is an extra role and responsibility at perhaps the most physically and emotionally demanding life stage she is likely to encounter. The decision to work at this time, therefore, is likely to be underpinned by a strong motivation. Women's motivations to work in the early years of their child's life fall into two broad categories: financial and personal.

FINANCIAL REASONS

Studies which have looked at the reasons women with pre-school aged children choose to undertake paid work consistently report that financial reasons are the primary motivation.[1, 14] Financial motivations may take a number of forms. A woman's income may be the sole income, as in the case of single mothers or an essential part of the total family income. For many women there is a pressure to work to maintain the standard of living achieved prior to the family as two comments taken from a study by Julia Brannen and Peter Moss illustrate:[3]

> *If I wasn't working about two weeks (each month) of my husband's salary would go on the mortgage. We wouldn't have a lot to live on and I am a one for buying clothes for the baby . . . we've accepted a certain standard of living and we are not really prepared to drop below it.*
> *Alice, 29, hospital pharmacy technician*

> *The house is considerably more expensive than the one we'd hoped to buy. If we'd got the other one I could have been off work a lot longer – probably the full six months and possibly could have given up work.*
> *Gillian, 32, executive officer in the civil service*

Lois Hoffman reports that between 55 and 90 per cent of women with young children, when asked why they work, will state 'money' as the prime reason.[14] She notes, however, that financial necessity or even supplementing family income may be a socially acceptable reason to give for working because society still holds the view that a mother's place is with her child. In support of this claim is the finding that many women when asked whether they would continue to work if they had enough money say that they would. One study found that exactly half of the mothers with pre-school aged children answered in this way and gave personal reasons for wanting to go out to work.[15]

Julia Brannen and Peter Moss report that working for financial reasons is more common among those employed in less well paid work such as clerical, secretarial and manual occupations.[3] However, it is also given as a reason, though not so frequently, by women in higher paid occupations. In their study 40 per cent of women in lower paid occupations said they worked for money and a further 33 per cent said they specifically worked to finance housing; a total of 73 per cent, this compares with 21 and 23 per cent, total 44 per cent, for those in well paid occupations. Women in well paid occupations were more likely to give personal reasons for working than those in lower paid occupations.

PERSONAL REASONS

The prime personal reasons given by women with young children returning to paid work are personal satisfaction, avoidance of household duties and maintenance of career. A major theme which emerges in studies of the motivation for paid employment among mothers of young children is that many of these women become disenchanted with the role of mother and housekeeper:

The achievement of giving birth is only briefly recognised. Many young mothers soon lose their own identity and come to be regarded (by themselves as much as others) merely as an extension of their children by day and their husbands by night. So the pressure on women today is to go back to work in order to *participate* in society and not simply for economic reasons.[16]

The writings of Ann Oakley in her books *The Sociology of Housework*, *From Here to Maternity* and *Women Confined* provide excellent examples of the frustrations of unpaid work in the home.[17-19] Although motherhood is rewarding, work in the home is never completed, the hours are long and the status accorded it low:

> *When I was working I used to come back here and get a tremendous kick out of doing housework. But now I am doing it every day, it really is the biggest bore of my life. I suppose it is because I can't do anything uninterrupted and I still can't get used to that. It takes a lot of effort.*
>
> *I used to read all the literature about having a baby, and really there is a tremendous halo of enjoyment – no one ever tells you about the hard work – no one tells you about how shattering it is to be doing it all the time, seven days a week . . . it's not all a super enviable state. It sounds awful because one has a child and she's super and beautiful and I wouldn't be without her either – to suddenly change from working – I'm thirty now – to suddenly find yourself doing housework all the time.[17]*
>
> *Juliet, 30*

Alongside the feeling of low status is a loss of identity:

> *I don't like the low status and I don't like the unsociable hours. This thing – the fact that society doesn't value it. It's the thing of 'just being a mother – just being at home.'[3]*
>
> *Clinical psychologist*

> *(I'm going back to work for) sanity (laughs) . . . I want to go back because of what I don't want to do.[3]*
>
> *Careers officer*

and independence:

> *When I was on unpaid leave I didn't have so much money. I had a slight guilty feeling about going out and spending money and enjoying myself.[3]*
>
> *Hospital administrator*

It may also be lonely and frustrating:

> *It can make you very lonely. If my husband wasn't around I wouldn't see anyone all day . . . And the frustration as well . . . you feel frustrated that you can't get on with all the work – And I mean you want to get on with your own interests and you can't do them.*[3]
>
> Alison, teacher

Going out to work in contrast provides a source of independence, and status, and a break from the frustrations of work at home.

For many women, particularly those in higher status occupations, paid work is challenging and a source of personal satisfaction and identity:

> *I love my child but I love my job too. I am a better person all round when I'm working – as a mother and partner as well – because although I am tired I am more stimulated and more stimulating to be with.*[6]
>
> Alice, 34, educational psychologist

> *Personal satisfaction is as important as anything else . . . I mean I enjoy my work. That is the main reason for going back – that I enjoy it.*[3]
>
> Teacher

> *I've got lots of exciting things to do. I enjoy what I am doing . . . I was quite excited about the challenge. It was really quite invigorating to be back and feel I could work again. I felt my old self.*[3]
>
> Clinical psychologist

Maintaining career is important. Some women express concern that if they do not return to work at least on a part-time basis they will lose sharpness of mind or lose touch:

> *I certainly felt my brain had gone out the window . . . I felt my attention span was so much less . . . eight months is a long time and my job is management.*[3]
>
> Senior physiotherapist

Things change fast in my profession. If I took too long out I would never get another job – I wouldn't have publications or grants for those years – and that is why universities want to employ you.[6]

Ilona, 35, University lecturer

Do the reasons for working vary according to the age at which a woman has her children? Evidence on this comes from the Australian Timing of Motherhood study (*see Table 9.4*) in which a comparison was made of early, average and late timing mothers according to their reasons for currently working.[6] No differences between the groups were found. For all groups the primary motive given was financial, with approximately half of all women giving this as their sole reason for working and between 30 and 40 per cent as one of a combination of reasons. The next frequent reason for early and late timing mothers was personal satisfaction, but for average timing mothers career maintenance ranked as the second most important reason. In this study late timing mothers were defined as being over 30. When the reasons for working given by women who were 35 or over were looked at separately a more distinct pattern emerged. Of this group only 12 per cent worked for financial reasons, but the majority, 63 per cent, worked for personal satisfaction and the remaining 25 per cent to maintain career. The number of women in this group was small but the findings suggest that women who become mothers over the age of 35 are more likely to return for personal rather than financial reasons.

Reasons for not returning to paid work

SOCIAL PRESSURES

Throughout history women's participation in the workforce has fluctuated according to society's needs. So, too, have the views about the 'rightness' or 'wrongness' of being a working mother. Since the Second World War and particularly since the influential work of John Bowlby, published in 1951, the view most prominent in societies like Britain and the United States is that the best carer for a child is his or her mother and, therefore, that to go out to work in the early years of a child's life is somewhat detrimental to his or her well-being.[20, 5] John Bowlby put forward the concept of 'maternal deprivation' which suggested that young children who were separated from their mothers in the early years of life did not develop a secure attachment to their mothers, were unable to establish good social relationships with others and were more likely to suffer poor mental health. This theory was originally based on observations of the behaviour of children who had experienced prolonged separation from their mothers, (children raised in institutions such as orphanages and hospitals), but it was extended to apply to children experiencing short separation, such as day-care, too. More recent work has questioned the applicability of Bowlby's theories to children raised within a family context.[5, 21] Nevertheless, Bowlby's ideas still remain influential in society today:

> *I don't know if I think* [going to work] *is right . . . I suppose inside myself I don't think it is right . . . I suppose it is because he is so little and you're so attached to him.*[3]
>
> Librarian, 24

Table 9.4. Reasons for returning to work for early, average and late timing of motherhood groups

Reasons for working	Early (%)	Average (%)	Late (%)	35+ (%)
Financial	42	47	49	12
Personal satisfaction	12	0	14	63
Career maintenance	0	11	6	25
Other	0	6	3	0
Combined financial and personal satisfaction	46	36	28	0

Source: Thorpe & Cinnamon, Australian Timing of Motherhood study[6]

Research studies report that a major reason given by women who do not go out to work in the early years of a child's life is concern that their absence will be bad for the child.[22-24] Professional women who opt not to work, in particular, have been reported as stressing a sense of duty to stay at home. The attitude of a woman's partner has also been found to be important. Some women feel pressured by their partners to remain at home after the birth of their child.[1] The absence of adequate day-care for children, perhaps reflecting society's view of working mothers, is also a possible deterrent to returning to paid work.[3,25]

PERSONAL MOTIVATIONS: THE REWARDS OF MOTHERHOOD

Motherhood, particularly when separated from general household duties, is a very fulfilling experience and many women feel that they can best enjoy their children by being at home full-time with their child in the pre-school years.[17] The rewards of motherhood are less tangible than those used to explain motivations for return to work (e.g. money, career) and have a greater emotional component:

> *Yes, I like looking after my child. I'd rather be at home with my child than at work – or anything else I could think of . . . I expected to find it rewarding but not quite as much as it is . . . Just the whole thing of seeing a person developing and somebody learning right from nothing to do things and be – and the amount of influence you have on this for good or bad.*[17]
>
> *Catherine*

> *I realize now that motherhood far surpasses other things like career and travel. I love being at home with my son, I wish that I had started having children earlier so that I could have more before I am 40.*[6]
>
> *Vivienne, 32, physiotherapist*

Lois Hoffman reports that women who decide to remain at home after the birth of their child not only find motherhood rewarding but enjoy the freedom and autonomy associated with not being in paid work.[14] This may be particularly so for women whose previous employment had been restrictive or unfulfilling.

Do the reasons for deciding not to return to paid work vary

according to the age of the mother? In the Australian Timing of Motherhood study across all timing groups personal choice, '*I prefer to stay at home*' was the most frequently given reason for staying at home. The proportion of women who gave this as their reason increased with the age of the mothers rising from 50 per cent in the early timing group to 84 per cent in the late timing group (*see Table 9.5*). When reasons given by 35-plus mothers were looked at separately it was found that a full 100 per cent said they stayed home through personal choice. Earlier timing mothers were more likely to report inability to find a job or inability to afford day-care; possibly reflecting the fact that they had lower status occupations and less well developed careers before having a child. The picture that emerges is that whether her decision is to become a full-time mother and homeworker or to return to paid work there is a greater element of personal choice for women having children over the age of 35.

Table 9.5. Reasons for not returning to work for early, average and late timing of motherhood groups

Reasons for not working	Early (%)	Average (%)	Late (%)	35+ (%)
Can't find job	11	0	0	0
Prefer to stay at home	50	69	85	100
Can't find child-care	0	0	0	0
Can't afford child-care	4	8	0	0
Other	35	23	15	0

Source: Thorpe & Cinnamon, Australian Timing of Mother study[6]

A woman who decides not to return to paid work opts to make a change of life role from income earner to that of primary carer for her child. While there are implications for the woman's own identity (discussed below), the issue of care for her child is resolved. For those who opt to return to paid work outside the home decisions about the care of the child have to be made.

Choosing day-care

Making decisions about day-care is seldom easy. Moreover, the major responsiblity for this decision is usually borne by the woman and not her partner.[3] The range of care arrangements made by women returning to work is huge but generally falls into four broad categories: family/friends, carer in the child's home ('nanny'), carer outside the home (childminder), and group care in a nursery. The choice made depends on five main factors: availability, cost, reliability, preference for single versus group care, and quality of carer.

COST

The least costly form of care is typically informal arrangements with family and friends who may or may not expect payment, while a carer in the child's own home is the most expensive option. All types of paid care are likely to account for a large proportion of a woman's earnings and, most commonly, payment for day-care is made from the woman's salary in dual income homes.[3] Clearly higher income earners, because they can afford it, have more choice about the type of care used. They are more likely to use formal care arrangements and, in Britain, more likely to opt for more expensive forms of carer – nannies or private nursery.[3]

AVAILABILITY

Choice of care is restricted by availability and for certain groups certain types of care are less available. Those who do not have relatives living near by, for example, will be unable to opt for informal care arrangements with their family. The availability of subsidized places is very limited in Britain, Australia and the US. Throughout Europe it varies with some countries, such as Denmark and France, having high levels of provision. Some women have workplace nurseries available to them though these are still relatively rare.

RELIABILITY

A woman returning to work needs to have the security that her day-care arrangements are reliable. Absences from work because of failed child-care arrangements are not generally acceptable to employers or to the women themselves.

You have got to be spotless, you can't afford to take a day off because of sick children, whereas a man possibly can, because no one would ask him, or for that matter blame him.[26]

Woman manager

Group care is typically the most reliable when the carer is considered. Illness of single carers such as childminders and nannies may prevent them working. An ill child, on the other hand, cannot be taken to a group setting and may result in a mother's inability to attend work. Informal arrangements, particularly if these are not paid may prove the least reliable and are very much dependent on the relationship between the carer, mother and child.

SINGLE VERSUS GROUP CARE

Reliability of group care is often set against a concern that it is 'not good for the child'. For some mothers the concerns about separation from the child lead them to prefer a 'mother substitute' with whom they can develop a relationship or attachment:

I wouldn't be happy with any form of group care because I want her to have as near a one to one relationship as she has with me.[3]

Senior laboratory technician

For others the fear that their role as mother will be usurped means that they prefer a group setting.

I feel I would mind the baby having a relationship with one other woman . . . I'm jealous I want my own to want me.[3]

Nurse

QUALITY OF CARERS

Control over the quality of carers in societies such as Britain and the United States are both variable and limited.[25, 27] There are greater controls over certain types of care. In Britain, for example, government regulations control the staff to child ratio and the qualifications of those in group day-care settings. These paid childminders must also register with local government authorities, but there is not similar control over minders in the child's own home (nannies). Informal arrangements are impossible to regulate in this way. Judgement of the quality of carer is left with the mother for those choosing these forms of care. For the former, qualifications, experience and personal references are the basis for making this decision while for informal arrangements the relationship between the mother and carer is the basis on which the mother must judge if the carer is acceptable.

What do women in general choose? The choice of day-care for women returning to work is different for those in professional, better paid occupations than for those in lower status less well paid occupations.[3] This is because the factors discussed above, particularly cost and availability, limit the range of choice open. Those in lower status occupations are more likely to use a relative or friend to care for their child while those in professional occupations are more likely to use formal care. A far higher proportion of professional women opt for private nurseries.[3]

What choices do 35-plus mothers make? There is no specific evidence concerning the choice of day-care made by later timing mothers, but two factors make it likely that they will chose formal care. Firstly, the social network of older mothers is typically different from that of younger timing mothers. Their friends are likely to be similarly professional women who work and their family less likely to live nearby. Moreover, parents or parents-in-law, who are often the carers for younger mothers may well be older and less suitable to care for a young child. Secondly, as they are often professional women who have higher incomes and more developed careers they can more often afford the costs of formal care and have greater choice in this respect.

The experience of returning to paid work

No matter how great a woman's commitment to returning to work, leaving a young child in the care of another is not easy. For many women separation from their child in the early days of return is stressful:

> *Everyone kept telling me how well I had got back into the swing of work so soon after having the baby (12 weeks), but underneath I was dying of grief – my heart was breaking – I hated leaving her.*
>
> *Alice, 34, educational psychologist*

> *Leaving him was a wrench. I am not sure if it was depression or what. Or whether it was a selfish sort of thing. I just missed him.*[3]
>
> *Assistant solicitor, 29*

With time women report that they get used to leaving their child:

> *I really felt in that first week as if my heart was breaking – leaving her. I thought 'I am never going to get over this.' But it's got easier now. It is a bit like a broken love affair, I suppose. It mends.*[3]
>
> *Teacher, 29*

After the initial wrench most women adapt to working and leaving their child; many report that they enjoy it though some 'feel guilty' about enjoying being away from their child. Guilt is also commonly expressed about leaving the child.[3, 26, 28]

Is there any evidence that day-care is bad for a child? A large number of studies in recent years have looked at the impact of day-care on the development and well-being of the child.[26, 29] The results of these studies, which have focused on formal day-care in group settings, are too many to discuss in detail here, however, in general, their findings are positive about day-care. They report that day-care is not in itself bad for a child: the quality of day-care is of key importance. There is no reason why a child in good quality care should not develop well and be well adjusted and there may even be some advantages. In this context it is also important to consider the alternative; care at home. The quality of care and stimulation provided for the child in the home setting is equally important for a child's development and well-being. Simply being cared for at home by a non-working mother does not guarantee that the child will develop well socially and intellectually. A mother unhappy with her life at home may not be the best carer. A woman's view of her own identity and life roles are important to her emotional well-being and this, in turn, will have an impact on her relationship with her child.

ᘒ

The impact of the multiple roles of motherhood and career

I feel career is hollow without the joy of some sort of 'family' and yet motherhood without anything else is a life unfulfilled.[6]
Jennifer, 35, teacher

Paid work as a source of stress

Women who return to paid work do not lose or reduce their responsibilities for care of the home or care of the children. Paid work is typically an additional role to that of mother and housekeeper. Studies of dual income couples prior to having children have found that although both partners will hold the egalitarian ideals that household chores should be shared, in reality the woman has a disproportionate share of household duties and takes the major responsibility for them.[28, 30, 31] Once children enter such families the additional responsibility of child-care does not mean that the woman loses some of her household responsibilities, but on the contrary her responsibility for household chores has been found to increase. Janice Steil and Beth Turetsky[31], for example, found in their study of dual income families in the United States that after the birth of a child not only did women acquire a greater share of household responsibility but they lost influence with a decreased role in decision making. The expectation that care of the home and the children is primarily the responsibility of a woman is one held not only by male partners and society in general, but also by the women themselves, as this quote from a study of women managers illustrates:[3, 32, 33]

> *I remember last week we were still at a meeting at 8 p.m. and one of the men said 'Oh excuse me, I must phone my wife and tell her I will be late for supper'. It made me very cross. Although my husband does cook, I think, as a woman, you should do most things in the house. Mind you, I hardly ever switch off and I get very, very tired.*[26]
>
> Business manager[26]

Women feel that they should be good employees, good house-keepers and good mothers and often express feelings of guilt because they perceive they are not carrying out their multiple roles well.[3, 28, 32] To compensate they forego leisure time. The same woman manager quoted above goes on to say

> *My major stress at home is definitely the children, and worrying that I am not a good mother. I was very, very upset when my little girl said to me, 'I know you won't have time, but I would like you to read me a story.' It was a Sunday morning as well! The fact that I work more through the lunch times compared with men at work is because the night before I was helping the children with homework and things. You just have to find ways of finding more time.*[26]
>
> Business manager[3]

and another similarly reports:

> *A potential source of stress which I have been able to keep at bay so far, is at the end of the day having to deal with the two children and playing fair by them and managing to switch modes, rather than putting my feet up and having a drink. I get little help from my husband.*[26]
>
> Research manager, mother of two children under 3 years[3]

Working mothers have been said to have 'role overload' and are undoubtedly stressed by the weight of responsibility and sheer physical work that they have to do.[28, 31, 34, 35, 36, 37] Some women deal with their multiple roles by adopting 'a woman's pattern of work'[28] and working part-time.[28] The consequence of this is invariably loss of status and reduced chance of promotion:

> *I know that it is disastrous (for my career to work part-time), and I know that it gives Phil an excuse to leave most of the hard work at home to me, but it is the only way I can manage right now.*[28]
>
> *Jane, physician*

Whether she works part-time or full-time the additional role of work after becoming a mother has been found to be stressful. Is work therefore 'bad' for a woman once she is a mother?

Paid work as a source of strength

Although going out to work as a mother of young children can be stressful, it can be, particularly for those in professional occupations, an important source of identity, independence and self-esteem.[34-36] In contrast, being out of paid work to be a full-time mother and housekeeper is accorded low status and may have a negative impact on a woman's self identity.[17-19] Pehaps reflecting these issues of identity and status is the consistent finding that women who do paid work have better health and those who do not are vulnerable to poor health especially depression.[34, 35, 37, 38]

One important element in the impact of work on the health of working mothers is whether she has choice in the decision to work. Ellen Hock and Debra DeMeis found that women who remained at home to care for their children out of personal choice did not have poor health profiles, and specifically did not experience symptoms of depression.[39] In keeping with previous findings, however, they found that women who stayed at home to care for children but who would have preferred to work were vulnerable to depression. In the light of the findings that women over 35 have greater choice in decisions about return to work it would seem that they are less likely to be adversely affected by a decision not to return to paid employment.

Paid work and particularly career development is, to a significant proportion of women who have their children over the age of 35, an important part of their reasons for their timing of motherhood and will also influence the role they take and their experience of motherhood. One late timing mother from the Australian Timing of Motherhood study felt very strongly about society's mixed messages of the importance of full-time motherhood, the low status accorded it, the importance of paid work and career and yet the failure to provide adequate child-care.[6] Though this mother's comments do not reflect the facts about risk to women of having children later (*see Chapter 5*) her concerns about the pressures of combining career and motherhood are very real. Women having children later have greater control over their choices about returning to paid work but for this group as much as any other it remains a difficult decision. We finish with her comments as a point for reflection:

> *I feel it is a great shame that women with careers are not encouraged to have children earlier – that is in their mid-twenties – with more child-care in the workforce and a loosening of the work and child-rearing situation so that both are symbiotic rather than conflicting. After 30, and especially late thirties, the risk of infertility, difficult pregnancies, disabled babies, birth and pregnancy problems are a lot greater and there often isn't the time biologically or 'chance' to fix these problems. A lot of women miss out on wanted children or have very troubled pregnancies all because career is seen as a first priority and incompatible with motherhood. I feel we are experiencing a reverse of the 1950s when having a baby before 25 was essential. Now under 30 is viewed as a non-career option designated for the uneducated suburban mums. All ages should be regarded as an option – child-care in the workforce is the way.[6]*
>
> *Jennifer, 35*

✺ 10 ✺

Older Mothers and Their Children: Are Older Mothers Better?

Women over 45 should not have babies.
No young child should have to cope with an elderly mum.[1]
Germaine Greer, academic and author, 1992

Older women 'have time to make children feel important'.[2]
Headline in the Independent, 4 January 1994

My mother was 43 when I was born . . . She was always grey-haired
when I knew her, and she looked older than all the other mothers. I
hated her coming to school events.[3]
Audrey Slaughter, magazine founder, editor and novelist, 1994

The older woman has more experience, has a better understanding of
people, she's wiser, her judgements are tempered with humanity in a
way that a younger woman's tend not to be . . . Because the older
woman is able to stand back (emotionally) to monitor and evaluate
herself, other people and events, I think she communicates some of her
own wisdom to her offspring.[4]
Sheila Rossan, psychologist, Brunel University

Popular attitudes towards older mothers

Today popular wisdom holds that motherhood is for women in
their twenties. The medical perspective on older mothers has
always emphasized the increased risks and problems that later

motherhood entails – risks for both mother and child and although less has been said in the media about the psychological aspects of later parenthood there often seems to have been a prejudice against older parents.[5] As this book has shown, the extent of the medical risks for women of 35 and over is probably much less than was once thought and, in reality, if a woman and her partner want children at this stage, and the choice is now or never, no woman need feel that the risks are too great. A woman in good health can still expect a happy outcome to a pregnancy.

As psychologists, our particular interest is in the experience of later motherhood for women themselves and for their children. Are older mothers different in their approach to child-care and in what ways does it make a difference for a child to have a 35-plus mother?

The title of this chapter poses the question: are older mothers better? Popular wisdom again would tend to stress the ageist view that older parents could never be better than younger ones. In an assessment of the psychological literature there are clearly some positive aspects to later parents *for their children* and we will discuss these in this chapter. In addition, the clearly problematic aspects will also be considered – in particular the likelihood for children that their parents will be old and infirm whilst the children are in young adulthood, and that the death of parents, perhaps before grandparenthood is achieved, is also more probable than for children of younger parents.

A major difficulty for us, in writing this chapter, is the dearth of well-designed research on older mothers and their children. There are very few research studies that have attempted to compare older mothers and their children with a younger comparison group. The few studies available are primarily concerned with the early stages of motherhood and focus on new babies and toddlers.[6-14]

There has been very little observational research on older mothers and their children – most existing studies are *retrospective* accounts. In these, women are asked to recall their experiences of having and raising children; women are not observed and interviewed at different stages as their children develop. What is needed is a *longitudinal* approach where individuals are followed over a number of years as their families grow up.

Most available research evidence and popular books on the topic of older mothers and their children comes from anecdotal evidence – accounts by individuals asked about being an older mother, or being a child of an older mother/parents.[5, 11, 15-24] Such accounts can highlight individual experiences but as the basis for making generalizations about such mothers and children they have two important flaws. Firstly, they provide no evidence on which to assess the extent to which each individual account can be seen as reflecting a more general experience. Secondly, these accounts come from individuals who have been asked to consider how age (their age, or that of their mother) might have influenced their experiences. Such questions might generate useful insights into the possible effects of age on motherhood or the experiences of having an older mother, but age may be used as an explanation for behaviour or experiences that in reality are not attributable to age. Age, like sex or race, is a convenient hook on which to hang explanations because it is a very obvious one. Differences may, in fact, be due to different life or learning experiences and it is vital to be able to distinguish between true age effects and other possible influences.

To put it briefly, the available evidence on older mothers and their children is very patchy and incomplete. Much more well-designed research is needed before we can paint a comprehensive picture – but we shall consider the evidence that is available in this chapter.

~

35-plus mothers and their babies

Enjoyment and pleasure

Iris Kern summed up her older motherhood research in the title of her paper '. . . an endless joy . . .' and her mothers were 'over-whelmingly favourable' in their assessment of the experience of having a later baby (86 per cent).[6] This very positive attitude was also found in the British study of 40-plus mothers.[9, 10] The 40-plus women felt that they had a great deal to give their baby and over 90 per cent recommended the experience to others.

Arlene Ragozin and colleagues found that the older mothers of pre-term babies showed greater pleasure in the overall parenting role than did younger mothers and she linked this to their greater commitment to parenting.[7] Walter reported that a higher percentage of late timing mothers ranked their children as their number one source of satisfaction than did early timing mothers.[2] Other research has shown that younger mothers stress the 'enormous sacrifices' of motherhood, whereas older mothers are more 'accepting' of their role.[25]

We cannot say how the experience of enjoyment and pleasure by the mother influences the situation for the child. It would seem to bode well but this needs to be investigated. However, not all studies reflect a *greater* level of enjoyment or satisfaction in later motherhood. The Australian Timing of Motherhood study found *no age-related* differences on these measures.[13]

Being patient and relaxed

When asked about the special qualitites that an older mother might have to offer her child, many women on the British study of 40-plus mothers referred to 'more patience and understanding' in answering this question.[9, 10] Most first-time mothers in this study felt that they would be more patient with their offspring as a mother at 40-plus than they would have been if they had given birth in their twenties. Having more patience was reported by just over half of those with one or more previous children; the majority of these mothers believed that they would be more relaxed at 40-plus than they were formerly. Less than half of the first-time mothers reported feeling that they would be more relaxed than a younger mother. Thus the older mother of a first child is more likely to have patience, whereas if she has other children her approach is more likely to be relaxed. As Shirley, aged 49, pointed out in Chapter 1 *'One is lazier and less bound by theories . . .'* This more easy-going approach she saw as an advantage for her later baby.

Emotional maturity

Both the American study by Iris Kern and the British study of 40-plus mothers reported that women felt that their own emotional maturity was a positive factor in their relationship with their baby and in their approach to child care.[6, 9, 10]

> *With maturity comes an increased appreciation of life, which enables an increased appreciation of the child . . .*
>
> *I'm far better able to accept him as himself . . .*[6]
>
> Two mothers from Iris Kern's study

In the British study of 40-plus mothers, four out of five of the first-time mothers believed that they had special qualities to offer their babies and '*a maturer outlook on life*' was stressed repeatedly.[9, 10]

Motherhood has always been viewed as 'one of the most challenging developmental tasks a woman faces during her life' and yet its meaning and significance for the individual woman varies with her own particular stage in life.[21] Ramona Mercer found this to be true for her sample of mothers but each age group approached the stage with entirely different perspectives.[8] Teenage mothers talked of motherhood making them feel good mentally, feeling important and having '*someone to grow up with me*'. Women in their twenties saw motherhood as making them '*a responsible adult member of society*', whilst those in their thirties and early forties felt that motherhood for them meant a lot of '*redefining of yourself*'; they felt complete having done all the other things that they wanted to do and were, as mothers, feeling '*a sense of sharing my life, a sense of posterity*'. It is clear that the older group saw motherhood less in terms of the gateway to maturity, but they nonetheless saw it as enabling them to foster and develop new facets of themselves.

Carolyn Walter suggests, from her study on the timing of motherhood, that one of the difficulties that a young mother will encounter is physical and emotional separation from her child 'because she herself is struggling with separation and individualisation in her adult life'.[21] It is clear that the degree to which a mother can allow her child independence may be influenced by the maturity (not necessarily the age) of the mother.

Maturity may be demonstrated in a number of ways: Ramona Mercer found that her older mothers scored more highly on the level of social and psychological development – and that thus age and maturity were linked.[8] In addition the older mothers were more flexible and they scored better or more adaptively on personality traits and childrearing attitudes. They showed high competency skills and scored better (in their own assessment) on handling an irritating child. Arlene Ragozin's research indicated that older mothers have a greater commitment to parenting and this can be viewed as a positive benefit for their children.[7]

Maternal responsiveness and caretaking

On a variety of measures of maternal responsiveness and behaviour, older mothers showed attributes that would seem to have positive benefits for children.

In the Australian Timing of Motherhood study older mothers responded more quickly to their crying baby by picking them up than did the younger mothers; they also took their infant out to more organized activities.[13] The study also found that the early timing mothers reported that motherhood was difficult although there were no age differences in how confident or relaxed mothers perceived themselves to be.

Arlene Ragozin's research showed that raised maternal age was linked with both increases in caretaking responsibilities and decreases in social time away from the babies.[7] This author noted that older women were better able to cope with 'the crises of pre-term delivery' and that an event such as a pre-term birth might bring into sharp focus any age-related differences in emotional maturity that might be less evident in studies of full-term babies and their mothers.

Breastfeeding

One aspect of a high commitment to motherhood may be the method of infant feeding chosen. Breastfeeding appears to be more common amongst older mothers: recent surveys in Britain show that raised maternal age is consistently associated with an increased incidence of breastfeeding.[26-28]

Iris Kern's sample of mothers all breastfed and in the British study of 40-plus mothers over two thirds of the mothers in the sample breastfed and breastfeeding extended for longer in the babies born after the age of 40 (in both parity groups) relative to the younger comparison group.[6, 9, 10]

In the Leicester Motherhood Project breastfeeding was also much more prevalent in older mothers.[14] All mothers in the 35-plus age group breastfed; the women who did not breastfeed were all from women in the younger age group (20–29).

Tiredness and health

Physical fatigue is often mentioned as a problem for the older woman with a new baby. Kern's mothers frequently noted the problem of physical exhaustion with '*several mothers reporting being tired much, if not all, of the time.*'[6] Ramona Mercer's older mothers reported greater fatigue than younger mothers one month after delivery. They also noted a lack of time because the change in their lifestyle was greater, in terms of reorganization, than that for younger women.

Some older mothers in the Leicester Motherhood Project linked age to tiredness:[14]

> *I'm more prone to being tired. I managed okay (with the first child) at 35. But now I'm over 40, I'm not so energetic.*
>
> Deborah, 40

> *You get tired more easily. You're more anxious because you know what can happen: youth is blind.*
>
> Suzanne, 37

The numbers of older and younger mothers reporting different levels of tiredness at the postnatal interview (approximately 17 weeks after the birth) did not differ: most women reported being 'moderately tired' or 'sometimes tired'. But at 13–14 months after the birth when women looked back over their first year after the birth 'extreme tiredness' was a problem for a higher proportion of older mothers than younger ones – 60 per cent of younger first-time mothers reported it compared with 77 per cent of the older first-timers.

The British study of 40-plus mothers found that whilst two thirds of first-time 40-plus mothers believed that tiredness was going to be a problem for them less than half of them said that this was actually the case. As tiredness is a 'normal' feature of early motherhood, indeed motherhood has been described as 'the most tiring job in the world', it is hard to assess the significance of this finding relative to a younger age sample.[29] It may be that older mothers explain their tiredness with a new baby in terms of age, whereas younger women do not – seeing tiredness as just one aspect of motherhood.

Jane Price found that the older mothers whom she studied varied a lot in relation to energy levels and tiredness; many believed that they had the same amount of stamina as in their twenties.[5] Breastfeeding is known to make mothers more tired than mothers of bottlefed babies and thus it may be that the higher commitment to breastfeeding evident amongst older mothers affects their tiredness levels.[30] Also, since older mothers are also more likely to return to paid work after their baby (*see Chapter 9*), both these factors may be relevant to tiredness reported in older mothers rather than simply their greater age.

In the Leicester Motherhood Project mothers were asked to report whether they had experienced a variety of symptoms in the first year or so after the birth of their baby. In addition to 'extreme tiredness' there were three other areas where the mother's age made a significant difference to the likelihood of the symptoms being reported. Significantly more older mothers reported pain in the legs; this was highest in 35-plus first-time mothers, 31 per cent reporting it, and lowest in younger first-time mothers amongst whom only 4 per cent reported leg pain.

Stress incontinence was a problem reported by women in all age and parity groups but whereas approximately half of the older mothers in both parity groups reported this only 12 per cent of younger first-time mothers and 30 per cent of those with previous children did so.

The occurrence of headaches in the first 13–14 months after the birth was also linked to the age of the mother but in this case significantly fewer older mothers experienced this problem. Indeed only 4 per cent of first-time 35-plus mothers reported headaches whereas 44 per cent of younger first-time mothers did so. Perhaps their lack of experience, both in life and infant care, makes coping with a new baby more stressful for them.

Emotional support

The importance of emotional support after the birth of a baby is of vital importance to the well-being of the mother as was noted in Chapter 7, and it is a key factor in reducing her risk of postnatal depression. Ramona Mercer found that a larger number of older mothers in her study reported having *more* emotional support during the first year after the birth, than did younger mothers, and they were more likely to report talking with others as a way of coping with difficult situations in mothering.[8]

A woman's own family might be viewed as one important source of support to a new mother, and in particular a woman's mother is often important at this time although this is not always so (*see Chapter 7*). In the Leicester Motherhood Project, despite women having fewer living parents in the older group, they were well supported emotionally and showed low rates of depression.[31] Ramona Mercer also found that older women less often described problems with their partner than did younger women and thus a settled and stable relationship with a partner might be expected to provide important emotional support for a new mother.[8]

The likelihood of depression

One of the hazards of motherhood is postnatal depression. Its incidence can be high – as we saw in Chapter 8 – but its link to raised maternal age is not established. This topic was considered in Chapter 8 and will only be summarized briefly here. The 'blues' has not been linked to raised maternal age;[32, 33] and neither has postnatal depression in most studies (*see Chapter 8*). However, two studies do indicate that there may be an increased risk amongst older first-time mothers.[33, 34] These studies indicate that two factors, Caesarean section delivery and lack of social support, may be important in its occurrence and as Caesarean section delivery has frequently been found to be more likely in older mothers (*see Chapter 5*) it seems fair to say that studies which do not compare age groups sharing similar levels of Caesarean sections or social support may be confounding age with these two factors.

Income and occupation

One of the most consistent findings in most of the studies of older mothers, especially first-time mothers, is the significantly higher family incomes found in this age group, as was discussed in Chapter 9. Women are more likely to be highly educated, and this makes the potential for a well-paid job greater.

Being an employed mother in the higher age groups had for both mothers and babies positive benefits in Ramona Mercer's research, since broadly speaking these women felt more positive feelings of love for their baby than non-employed women in the older age group.[8] The employed women's babies scored higher on the growth and development factor – unlike the babies of younger women where employed mothers' infants scored lower. Thus the effect of employment on motherhood, in this respect, was more positive for older than younger mothers. Ramona Mercer found that juggling paid work and motherhood was a major concern for a higher proportion of older mothers relative to younger women and it was a significant source of stress in the short-term. However, in the long-term paid work was *better* for the mothers' health.[35]

Feelings about the maternal role

Despite the evidence that women feel great joy and pleasure in later motherhood, Mercer reported that older mothers felt the least amount of gratification with the maternal role relative to the younger age groups.[8] One factor relevant to this may be the lack of experience in caring for infants that older mothers appear to have, compared with younger ones. Mercer suggests that highly educated women '*having high achievement orientation less often met their own expectations*' as far as the maternal role was concerned. Perhaps a woman who has been a high achiever in her career sets a very high standard for herself in motherhood which she may find hard to meet – at least in the early stages of motherhood.

♈

35-plus mothers and their children growing up

Older mothers of babies seem to have a number of positive attributes to offer in the way they relate to, and care for, their babies. Fatigue may be less of a problem than is often supposed, being common in most age groups, and there is evidence to suggest that older mothers have a good emotional support network, and are flexible and adaptive in dealing with a new baby. So do these positive qualities endure in coping with a toddler, a child and later an adolescent?

At the start of this chapter we noted several negative comments about the embarrassment that a grey-haired mother may engender in her 'later' child. Germaine Greer writes that this is something with which no child should have to cope, but perhaps set against other qualities this problem can be seen in perspective.[1]

Several of the studies reported in the previous section did not extend the research on having an older mother beyond babyhood. This applies to Ramona Mercer's research and that of Iris Kern for instance.[8, 6] The Leicester Motherhood Project will be investigating the children of the study later in their development (at age four) but children involved in this research are only just out of babyhood.[14] Earlier research studies suggested that older mothers may have a different way of approaching the care of their children and we shall now consider these findings.

Childrearing attitudes and practices

As we have noted older mothers have a reputation for being more patient with their babies and this attribute is emphasized by Andrew Yarrow's *Latecomers* in recalling their parents.[11] Similarly their maturity is viewed very positively by some of those he interviewed. *'People who have reached a plateau in their lives and aren't striving for greater glory have more time to love their children'* was how one woman put it; she linked maturity with an ability of parents to give love more freely. Yarrow also finds that older parents are more likely to foster independence, something that may be harder for the younger parent to do. Other researchers have also found that older mothers discourage dependency and encourage verbalization in their children.[36]

Robert Sears and colleagues in a research study in the 1950s found that the age of the mother influenced her approach to controlling or disciplining her children.[37] Younger mothers were 'somewhat more severe' in their treatment of young children. They also seemed to be more irritable in that a higher percentage were quick to punish, and more used physical punishment in controlling children. Ridicule was also more often used by the younger mothers. Sears' research investigated 379 mothers aged 24 and over (median age 33.5 years). A more severe approach to toilet training was also found amongst the younger mothers but Sears was more cautious in linking this solely to age, believing that this finding was more heavily influenced by mothers' social class; with working-class mothers showing greater severity in this respect.

In the British study of 40-plus mothers no differences were found between the two parity groups (first versus later born) in relation to discipline, routines and eating habits; nor did the treatment of the later babies differ from those of the infants born earlier in their mother's lives (on average in their twenties).

Thus, where differences are found between mothers of different ages these clearly *favour* the attitudes and practices of older women.

Intellectual development

One finding that has been shown to be positively linked to raised maternal ages is children's intellectual development. Arlene Ragozin and colleagues report this and note that: 'consistent results have been obtained from studies of different countries, races, social classes, and child ages.'[7] This relationship between maternal age and a child's IQ is evident even when the researchers have controlled for potentially confounding variables such as education and social class. For example, in a study of over 1500 young men carried out in the Netherlands, great care was taken to control for social class and birth order; the researchers, Patricia Zybert and colleagues, found a significant positive correlation between IQ and maternal age at birth of child.[38] Males came from two-child families and the relationship held for both first or second-born children. The reason for this effect is not entirely clear but may be related to maternal attitudes and behaviour which have beneficial effects on children. It has already been noted that older mothers encourage verbalization more and allow children more independence than younger mothers. Perhaps factors such as these, together with the greater commitment to parenthood often reported in studies of older parents – and noted particularly amongst first-time mothers by Arlene Ragozin and colleagues – play a contributory role in enhancing intellectual development; certainly it seems unlikely that age per se can be the cause.[7]

Financial security

Yarrow's account also highlighted the great financial security of many older parents and, whilst all will recognise that money does not take the place of love and care, its availability obviously can reduce the stresses and strains of day-to-day living that can have a major impact on the lives of parents and children.[11] In studies such as that by Mary Boulton it has been shown to be an important factor in releasing women from some of the drudgery that was once a major part of a mother's work.[39] Without being mercenary its role should not be underestimated in improving the lot of children. Sheila Rossan sums up some of the benefits:[4]

> In general, older couples are more financially secure than younger ones, so there aren't as many stresses related to finances – they have more resources to provide for the child.
> And:
> An older man has more time to spend with his children because he is more established.

The generation gap

The larger than usual general gap was felt to have an impact on the 'family climate' by Yarrow's latecomers.[11] Yarrow notes that 'later born children often lamented that their parents were emotionally distant, serious, and formal.' Informality and spontaneity was also often reported to be lacking and life seems to have been a more serious business for Yarrow's latecomers. As one woman recalled: '*It would have been nice to have a little more humour in my childhood.*'

It is of interest that their comments are not reflected in the assessment of older mothers in more recent research, where, on the whole, they appear to be more flexible than younger ones and more responsive and sensitive – at least in the studies of maternal behaviour in relation to babies. It may be, as Yarrow himself points out, that there are major cohort differences which influence each generation as they become a parent at whatever age.

Yarrow notes that children and young people of the more permissive 1960s may be quite different in their attitudes to offspring than the generation either before, or after them, where in both cases somewhat less permissive attitudes prevailed. Studies of age effects must take these differences into account. Yarrow's respondents do, however, frequently comment that parents were more serious or lacking in humour than they perceived other, younger parents to be, but Yarrow's work does not enable us to establish whether these qualities are due to age or to personality factors which those parents may have had *independent* of age.

Attitudes to the greater generation gap produced a variety of reactions. For some it fuelled rebellion in adolescence whereas others found it harder to rebel. Some said that they tried to rein in emotions so as not to upset their *'apparently-more-vulnerable older parents'*. Parents' old-fashioned and out-dated attitudes and opinions were often commented on. Again the extent to which these reactions would be significantly different from children of younger parents is impossible to assess from this study and we should be cautious in our interpretation of the significance of the findings.

The large generation gap between parents and their children can be viewed as advantageous by some children: *'I was never in competition with my parents' ambitions and desires'*, was how one of Andrew Yarrow's respondents described this. The father who always competes with his son in sports for instance, or the mother who competes with her daughter and likes to be mistaken for an older sister, are both examples of parents who lack the maturity to take a back seat. Perhaps older parents are no more mature than younger ones but simply have to face the fact that there is 'no contest' on looks and physique, or perhaps they just feel no need to compete. Whatever the reason the result may be beneficial for their children.

PARENTS LOOKING OLDER

One aspect of having older parents is, obviously, that they look older – indeed they may even look like the grandparents of children born to younger women and men as has already been noted (*see Chapter 1*: Shirley's account). Audrey Slaughter's comments at the start of this chapter show that she felt keenly about her mother's grey hair and '*hated her coming to school events*'.[3] It is obvious that women who have babies after 35 can also be grandparents simultaneously. One mother in the British study of 40-plus mothers had a gap of 28 years between her two children (one was born when she was 18, the other at 46).[9, 10]

Looking like a grandmother seems to be viewed, by some, as something of an insult to women. In the 1980s, the British Medical Association published a free manual for expectant mothers in which a section on 'Mature Mothers' warned about the likelihood of being mistaken for grandmother at the school gate.[40] Presumably the assumption here was that this is a blow to the self-esteem against which an older mother must brace herself. That it might be seen as a compliment does not seem to have been considered. In the British study of 40-plus mothers women were asked, '*Have you ever been mistaken for your child's grand-mother?*'[9, 10] Nearly one third had been (28 per cent of first-timers and 34 per cent of women with more than one child) and most were amused by the mistake.

Of course it's all very well for the mothers to be amused but what of their children? Children of later timing parents saw no disadvantages, concerning their parents' age, to themselves or to their parents according to Marjorie Gutman, reviewing the psychological aspects of delayed child-bearing.[41] Indeed she goes on to point out that children of some early timing parents wondered, as they reached adulthood, if their parents had been ready for them and thought that it might have been better for them if their parents had waited before starting a family.

The issue of grey hair may be of embarrassment to some children but its importance is hard to assess. A development of the argument might be that children of plain or ugly or fat or disabled parents may also feel embarrassment when they see them at the school gate. Parents can be a source of embarrassment for children whether they are of younger, average or older parents. Perhaps learning to cope with this is one import-ant aspect of children's development, not a justification for restricting the rights of adults of all sizes, shapes and ages to reproduce. In an ageist society it is no surprise if children's values reflect those of the adults in it – perhaps the adults' views on this issue need to be reassessed?

Being an only child

Being an only child is a disease in itself.

It would be best for the individual and the race that there be no only children.[42]

Being an only child is widely viewed as a 'bad thing'. Indeed in one research study the second most common reason for having a second child was to prevent the first one from being an only child.[40] Clearly the 'spoiled brat' in the West, and the 'little emperor' image in the East appear widely to influence couples when thinking about whether or not to have another child.[42, 43] But, as we saw in Chapter 1, not all women are certain that they want more than one child.

If a woman delays parenthood until after 35 what are her chances of having an only child? Will the baby be her first and last delivery? Martin Blum argues, however, that this view is erroneous; he found that more than a third of mothers aged 35 or more at their first delivery had more than one pregnancy and delivery during the five year period of the study.[44] In the British study of 40-plus mothers approximately ten per cent of mothers had more than one child in their forties.[9, 10] Thus for those delaying motherhood until their mid-thirties there is no reason to assume that a second child cannot be produced.

Obviously as women get older the chances that their first child will be their last increase. In a society where 'onlies' are generally not felt to be at an advantage this could be viewed as a potential hazard of delayed motherhood (whether voluntarily or otherwise). And it is one that can cause considerable heartache as the following comment shows:

Before I had my son, I had begun to feel I would have to come to terms with not having children, and felt I could cope. Now I have a child it's almost impossible to come to terms with not having any more children, to the extent that it has spoilt some of the enjoyment when my son was younger, being so preoccupied by fertility treatment (IVF etc.)[45]

Naomi, age 50, was awaiting egg donation at the time. She had spent twenty years trying to have children and in addition to the birth of her son, at the age of 42, she had had three miscarriages. She had abandoned hope of a second baby as her periods became scanty in her late forties and sought treatment with donor eggs.

On a more positive note, mothers of only children and those who are only children themselves may be relieved to discover that in a large review of the only child literature Toni Falbo and Denise Polit found that:[42]

Only borns were found to surpass all others except firstborns and people from two-child families on achievement and intelligence. They also surpassed all non-only borns, especially people from families with three or more children, in character and they surpassed all non-only borns, especially those from large families, in the positivity of the parent-child relationship. Across all developmental outcomes, only children were found to be indistinguishable from firstborns and people from small families.

These authors sum up by saying that their analysis contradicts the theoretical notions that only children are either deprived or unique. Indeed they suggest that enhanced parental attention, and the anxiety that is characteristic of new parents when coping with their first (or only born) is an important factor in their greater achievement, motivation and intelligence.

Finally it should also be borne in mind that siblings at any age are not an unmixed blessing. Having a sibling is no guarantee of having a friend and ally – jealousy, rivalry and even hatred can also be part of such a relationship.[46]

Children's long-term health and well-being

In Chapter 5 the link between raised maternal age and a few health problems and psychological disorders was noted.[47-50] The reasons for these particular associations are not known and we can only conclude that more research is needed on this topic before we can shed light on maternal age and subsequent health and psychological well-being in children.

ↄ

35-plus mothers and their adult children

We have already commented on the lack of well-controlled studies on the offspring of older parents and thus evidence for the impact of later motherhood – as their children enter adulthood – is scarce. It is chiefly based on reports from parents such as those in the 40-plus mothers study and on evidence from studies such as that by Andrew Yarrow.[9, 10, 11]

The mother's perspective

The research on British 40-plus mothers led, unexpectedly, to a large number of responses from women well beyond the child's age requirement specified in the letters of advertisement.[9, 10] In the latter, we requested that anyone who had had a baby in the last five years and who was 40 or over at the time of the birth should contact us. Thirty-eight women replied who had had their 40-plus child 21 or more years before the specified date of 1 November 1988. These women, all of whom were in their sixties or more, wanted to tell us of their experiences – and in general they felt that it had been a most positive one for them and their 'latecomer'. Volunteer samples such as this one, or that of Yarrow's, tend to be those who have polarized views and in our case these views were favourable.

Women were asked to rate on a five point scale from strong

agreement to strong disagreement a series of statements frequently made about older mothers and their children. Over half of these women agreed strongly that, '*a mother's age makes no difference to the child; attitudes and feelings are more important*'. Only eight per cent disagreed, or disagreed strongly. Nearly 60 per cent felt that for adult children the large generation gap does not matter and in a further question only 16 per cent believed that the large generation gap had always been a problem. Nearly half strongly disagreed with the latter statement. Over half agreed with the statement, '*I feel that I had a unique and special relationship*' with their child (born after 40). On the negative side, 45 per cent worried about dying before their 'late' baby grew up, and 24 per cent agreed that '*I often wish that I had completed my family when I was younger.*'

Across the whole sample of mothers over forty, over two thirds would recommend 40-plus motherhood and 60 per cent felt that the experience of having a later baby had given them '*a zest for life*'. Nearly half felt that it may have increased their life expectancy. Thus for many it was a most positive and invigorating experience.

> *I'd advise any woman to have a child later on in life. It's the best thing you can do.*[51]
>
> Tracy Dawson, whose husband was the late British comedian
> Les Dawson, on having a baby after 40

These glowing accounts put the case in favour of later babies; perhaps 'better late' in both the senses considered at the start of the chapter, but is this response echoed by their children?

The offspring's perspective

Andrew Yarrow's latecomers present a range of views, some positive, some negative – in Yarrows own words: 'it is rarely a neutral matter.'[11] His research indicated that people felt strongly one way or the other. However, as pointed out earlier, research of this type from samples recruited by advertisement generally produces those who have strong views and those who wish to express them – those who feel neutral on the subject simply do not respond and until research has a representative sample of children of older parents it is not possible to have an accurate perspective on the children of older parents.

Key issues for adult children of older parents, according to Yarrow, centre around 'losses'. He talks of 'youth foreshortened' and 'facing mortality' – plus the likelihood of becoming the caregiver to ageing parents when still young and contemplating parenthood themselves. Some of Yarrow's respondents made life choices that were obviously influenced by their parents' ages. '*I had my five children before I was twenty*,' one commented '*Deliberately!*' Another declared, '*To this day I actually get angry when I see someone over thirty who is going to have a baby.*'

Of Yarrow's group, 66 per cent of those surveyed said that their parents' ages influenced their feelings about what is the best time to have a child and although Yarrow notes that some said it was both right and beneficial to be and have older parents, 'about twice as many' believed that it is better for the child if parents have children earlier in life. One unexpected aspect of having older parents is the research finding that girls of older parents menstruate earlier than those with younger parents.[52] In a very real sense one aspect of youth is foreshortened.

Children of older parents may be less likely to have grandparents or if they have, then their grandparents will be older. The extent of this problem, of course, varies with the actual age of parents and is likely to be more pronounced in relation to grandfathers than grandmothers. In the Leicester Motherhood Project, mothers aged 35 and over when the target child of the study was born had fewer living parents than mothers aged 20–29 but this effect was much more marked for fathers, many more of whom had died.

Life expectancy today is much greater than it was in earlier times. Today in the UK a female's life expectancy at birth is 78.5 years and a male's is 73 years.[53] At the turn of the century these figures were markedly different – at birth, life expectation was 47.8 years for females and 44.1 years for males, increasing up to the age of 62.6 and 60.2 years respectively if they achieved the age of 15.[54] Thus the likelihood of having grandparents in 1900 would have been much less than it is currently for all children. Having living grandparents has become the expectation of all children today but this was not always so.

It should not be forgotten that set against this negative aspect of older parents is the positive aspect of the likelihood of a more stable relationship between older parents. Divorce rates have increased greatly since the mid-1960s and in Western Europe the expectation is that about one third of recent marriages can now expect to end in divorce.[53, 55] Children from such families have to cope with the loss of a parent (from the family home) and many will lose contact with one of their parents, usually the father. 'In Britain and America, 40 per cent of children never see their father at all after a divorce.'[56] Losing contact with a parent also means, in most cases, losing contact with one set of grandparents too, as well as all the other family members. As divorce rates are higher in the younger age groups, it would appear that the problem of separation and loss of a parent, and the associated grandparents, may be a key issue for a significant number of children from homes in which divorce has occurred.

The increased stability found in the relationships of older parents may be viewed as a clearly positive aspect for a child of such a family when set beside the issue of raised divorce rates in younger couples. From the child's point of view having two parents, whatever their age, may be a lot more preferable to losing one via divorce. Losing a much loved parent or grand-parent through death may be less damaging psychologically than losing one after the distress and anguish that often precedes a divorce, and the increased risk of total loss of contact with that parent soon after divorce.

Berry Brazelton, the Harvard paediatrician, has remarked,

> Older parents should convey that their children should feel lucky to have older, successful parents rather than tortured, searching, younger ones.[11]

Perhaps older parents have found what the young are searching for and have an aura of contentment about them that may be lacking in more youthful parents who have a higher risk of divorce.

༊ঌ

How old is too old?

Then Abraham fell upon his face and laughed, and said in his heart, shall a child be born unto him that is an hundred years old? And shall Sarah that is ninety years old bear?

The Bible, *Genesis, 17:17*

For Sarah conceived, and bore Abraham a son.

The Bible, *Genesis, 21:2*

The chief aim of this book has been to explore the facts about later or delayed motherhood, and also to explore the psychological aspects of this topic for both mothers and children. We have dealt primarily with children born to their biological mothers – the mothers, half of whose genes they share, and who bore them in pregnancy. Such older mothers are currently in their thirties and forties, but a few will be in their fifties too – as birth statistics show. Chapter 2 reported a recent birth to a grandmother of 59 and past reports indicate that 'natural' births may occur at even greater ages (*see Box 2.1 in Chapter 2*). Today older motherhood includes a very new type of mother – the woman who can give birth to a baby who does not share her genes – a baby who is the result of egg donation. Thus any discussion of later motherhood must now include those to whom this new treatment applies. Such women are not necessarily old – egg donation can be used for women who do not have their own eggs. Women with Turner's syndrome (lacking one X chromosome, referred to in Chapters 1 and 2), for example, may seek such treatment when young because they are known to be sterile.

There are now two dimensions to the age question in relation to having babies: the first is concerned with the issue of whether there is an age beyond which a woman should not try to become pregnant and have a baby (by whatever means), and the second is concerned with the ability of women, as they get older, to mother children effectively. These questions are often posed – both in the media and in academic journals. The *Lancet*, a well known British publication, discussed the age issue in a recent paper entitled 'A right to reproduce'.[57] Can we answer the question 'How old is too old?' and if we can is it a moral question for each individual to consider or is it one that should be legally defined?

Motherhood in later life

Part of this book has been concerned with women's qualities if they become an older mother: how does such a woman do the job of mothering after the age of 35. The research that is available indicates that though she may be different, in some ways, from her younger counterpart she is certainly not any less good as a mother. Indeed there are a number of studies that indicate that she has positive qualities that make her, in some respects, a better mother than a younger woman.

All women who have had children retain their role as mother for the rest of their lives. Their skills as they get older are honed by years of experience with their children, grandchildren and great grandchildren. The value of experience in caring for babies and children should not be underestimated. Some women who have a later addition to their family, perhaps years after their first children were born, find an enormous satisfaction and joy in their 'late' baby or 'caboose' baby.

Today, with the availability of abortion in most countries, few late babies need be unwanted babies. We know that abortion statistics tend to be very high amongst those over forty (varying between 40 to over 50 per cent in the last 10 to 15 years), but for those who do not choose this option it is likely that most will actively 'want' their later baby. The very late detection of a pregnancy, or strong moral or religious feelings against abortion may be exceptions here. Being wanted is viewed as one of the most important aspects of successful motherhood and thus most later babies will fit into this category.

One well-known British 50-plus mother, Kathleen Campbell, was advised to have an abortion and chose not to. She recalls:

> *The doctors thought it was the menopause when I went to them 13 weeks gone ... And when the test showed I was pregnant, they tried to persuade me to have an abortion.*[58]

Her child, though a surprise, was clearly wanted. It is fair to say that there is insufficient research on older motherhood to be able to comment on mothers giving birth in their fifties and later. The advent of babies by egg donation may increase research in this field but to date we can only look at other forms of evidence.

The older mother research available for 'younger' age groups is in many ways very positive about what older women have to offer. Other evidence comes from foster mothers and adoptive mothers who provide care in their fifties and older. Martin Shaw, in a review of 'substitutes' – those who are not the biological mother – reports that women can be very effective as mothers in later life.[59] Foster mothers are typically older women and in many parts of the world (oriental countries, for example) it is the grand-mother who cares for the children whilst the mother and father of the children undertake paid work. Adoption societies often have age limits from about 30 upwards, beyond which people become ineligible to adopt. These limits are wholly arbitrary and are certainly not based on women's and men's abilities as parents.

The weight of evidence available can be summed up thus: the competence of women as mothers after 35 is certainly no worse, it is equal to or possibly even somewhat better than younger mothers. It differs in some ways but there is no evidence to suggest women cannot mother effectively later in life. It is prob-ably also worth noting that if there was evidence to suggest that older women were slightly less capable, such evidence would best be used, in our view, to assist older women to become better mothers rather than to prevent them from having children, or oblige them to terminate a wanted pregnancy.

Egg donation in later life

If mothers are capable of mothering, but not capable of having their own infant, genetically, is it right to set age limits on this form of treatment? Fertility specialists such as Severino Antinori, in Italy, Mark Sauer in the US, and Ian Craft in Britian appear not to think so.[60, 61, 62] Mark Sauer comments[61]

> I don't think the pain of infertility is age-dependent. I think it's the same: I see it in their faces at 55, I see it in their faces at 25. If a woman who's 50 years old comes to me with that need, with that desire, and she has her own personal reasons, and I can help her as a doctor, then that's my challenge and that's my choice!

> I'm most concerned about the prejudice that I see towards ageing women both in society in general and in my medical colleagues, who presume that what we're doing is unethical and immoral.

> If it's OK for a man – and we have men coming in here with their second and third wives who can no longer produce sperm – if it's fine to use donor sperm for his young wife, why isn't it OK for the 55 year-old woman if she wants to have a 25 year old husband?

Severino Antinori believed that the birth to a 62 year-old woman, Rosanna Della Corte, marked the 'rebirth of the women'. On the day her baby was born he remarked:

> Today is a great day in Italy for women, individual liberty. To want to have a child is a personal choice and to be able to have it at any age is now possible.[60]

And concerning an age limit for such treatment he commented:

> It is clear that there must be a limit but that limit should be the woman's clinical condition.

As we saw from Ian Craft's comments in Chapter 4 he also argues that each case must be decided on its merits.[62] A range of factors need to be considered but these are essentially the business of the woman, her partner and the medical practitioner whom she consults, just as any younger woman thinks about these issues before a planned pregnancy.

The British Medical Association has expressed a range of conflicting views on this issue but more recently it, too, had indicated that age on its own should not be a bar to fertility treatment of this type.[63] The essential point is, should a decision to have a baby, even with medical treatment, be outside the control of the woman and her partner – especially when no constraints, or pressures of any kind, are placed on men as far as older fatherhood is concerned? That men can do it 'naturally' takes not one iota of responsibility away from them – as fathers.

Motherhood after 50 should neither be encouraged nor discouraged – in our, the authors, opinion. It is a personal matter, as it is at any age. It behoves all would-be parents to consider what they can offer their future child and to try to ensure that they can provide the love and care that is essential to health and well-being. The decision to become a later-life mother, with egg donation, does not rest solely with the parents because it involves fertility treatment. But, should not the decision to provide that treatment also be a matter for the individual doctor, with the woman and her partner, and not be a matter that is prescribed by some medical authority or law?

~

Conclusions

The old pearl-oyster produces the pearl

Chinese proverb

Although older motherhood is on the increase, research on the subject is relatively scarce. However, the evidence from those studies available indicates that older women have much to offer their children. The problems associated with having an older mother, in terms of feeling conspicuous amongst friends with younger parents, will diminish naturally as more people opt for later motherhood.

In our own study of 40-plus motherhood, most of the women taking part agreed that there was an ideal age for motherhood, but there was no consensus on when that age was.[9, 10] Responses ranged from '*it depends*' (on personal factors appropriate to the individual) to times in a woman's twenties or thirties to '*every age*'. The latter view was summed up by one mother of many children who answered the question by saying

I don't know – I have been 17, 18, 20, 24, 27, 31, 34, 36 and 43, and felt OK with all of them.

In research on later motherhood, most older women feel that having a baby later in life is a very positive experience. Such women feel that they have a lot to offer their 'later' child and are unconcerned about the larger than average generation gap. More research is needed on children's responses to later motherhood and two of the authors, Julia Berryman and Kate Windridge, are currently engaged in this. Research of this kind needs to be designed to enable comparisons to be made between children of older and younger parents. Our research will explore these comparisons and we hope to be able to tease out what the effects on children are of having older parents. Until that research is complete, we can only conclude that to date the available evidence on later motherhood – for both mothers and their children – is reassuring.

Today's older mothers have many positive qualities to offer their children and no child of an older mother need feel disadvantaged. The situation is one of 'swings and roundabouts', there are good and bad points; such mothers are certainly no worse than average age mothers, indeed as some research studies have shown they may be even better.[4]

References

2: Who has Babies after 35?
Facts and Figures

1. *Birth Statistics, 1987.* (1989). Review of the Registrar General on births and patterns of family building in England and Wales. Series FM1, no. 16. London: HMSO.
2. *Birth Statistics, 1992.* (1994). Review of the Registrar General on births and patterns of family building in England and Wales. Series FM1, no. 21. London: HMSO.
3. *Advance Report of Final Natality Statistics, (1988).* (1990). Monthly Vital Statistics Report: Final Data from the Nation Center for Health Statistics (1990), *39* (4). Supplement. 1–6 (see page 2).
4. Berkowitz, G.S., Skovron, M.L., Lapinski, R.H. & Berkowitz, R.L. (1990). Delayed childbearing and the outcome of pregnancy. *The New England Journal of Medicine, 322* (10), 659–63.
5. Thorpe, K.J. & Cinnamon, J. (1992). The Timing of Motherhood. Unpublished research report. University of Queensland, Australia.
6. Laslett, P. (1977). Characteristics of the western family considered over time. *Journal of Family History, 2* (2), 89–115.
7. May, R.M. (1978). Human reproduction reconsidered. *Nature, 272,* 491–95.
8. Gosden, R.G. (1985). *Biology of Menopause: The Causes and Consequences of Ovarian Ageing.* London: Academic Press.
9. Tanner, J.M. Cited in R.M. May. (1978). Human reproduction reconsidered. *Nature, 272,* 491–95 (see page 492).
10. Short, R.V. (1976). The evolution of human reproduction. *Proceedings of the Royal Society of London, 195,* 3–24.
11. Gray, R.H. (1976). The menopause – epidemiological and demographic considerations. In R.J. Bearch (ed) *The Menopause.* Lancaster: MTP Press.

240

12. Khaw, K.T. (1992). Epidemiology of the menopause. *British Medical Bulletin, 48* (2), 249–61.

13. Maroulis, G.B. (1991). Effect of aging on fertility and pregnancy. *Seminars in Reproductive Endocrininology, 9* (3), 165–175 (see page 116).

14. Eaton, J.W. & Mayer, A.J. (1953). The social biology of very high fertility among the Hutterites: The demography of a unique population. *Human Biology, 25* (3), 206–264 (see quotations on pages 206–7, 244).

15. Flinn, M. (ed). (1977). *Scottish Population History: From the 17th Century to the 1930s.* Cambridge University Press.

16. Dalen, P. (1977). Maternal age and incidence of schizophrenia in the Republic of Ireland. *British Journal of Psychiatry, 131,* 301–305.

17. *Demographic Yearbook, 1986.* (1988). United Nations: New York.

18. *Social Trends.* (1994). London: HMSO.

19. *Birth Statistics, 1991.* (1993). Review of the Registrar General on births and patterns of family building in England and Wales. Series FM1, no. 20. London: HMSO.

20. Wilkie, J.R. (1981). The trend towards delayed parenthood. *Journal of Marriage and the Family, 43* (3), 583–91 (see page 583).

21. Rindfuss, R. Cited in Harker, L. & Thorpe, K. (1992). 'The last egg in the basket', Elderly primiparity–A review of findings. *Birth, 19* (1), 23–30.

22. Cohen, B. Cited in Harker, L. & Thorpe, K. (1992). 'The last egg in the basket', Elderly primiparity–A review of findings. *Birth, 19* (1), 23–30 (see page 24).

23. Kern, I. (1982). '. . . an endless joy . . .': The culture of motherhood over 35. *Papers in the Social Sciences, 2,* 43–56.

24. Berryman, J.C. & Windridge, K.C. (1991). Having a baby after 40. I: A preliminary investigation of women's experience of pregnancy. *Journal of Reproductive and Infant Psychology, 9,* 3–18.

25. Berryman, J.C. & Windridge, K.C. (1994). Leicester Motherhood Project. Unpublished findings. University of Leicester, UK. (This study is not yet complete, analysis of data is in progress.)

26. Fleissig, A. (1991). Unintended pregnancies and the use of contraception: changes from 1984 to 1989. *British Medical Journal, 302,* 147.

27. Frankel, Steven A. & Wise, Myra J. (1982). A view of delayed parenting: some implications of a new trend. *Psychiatry, 45* (3), 220–25.

28. Welles-Nystrom, B.L. & de Chateau, P. (1987). Maternal age and transition to motherhood: prenatal and perinatal assessments. *Acta Psychiatrica Scandinavia, 76* (6), 719–25.

29. *U.S. Bureau of Census, Statistical abstract of the United States: 1993,* (113th edition), (1993). Washington, DC.

30. Illman, J. (1993). . . . and baby makes two. *Guardian*, 18 February.
31. Hubbard, F. (1994). Women who want the baby but not the man. *Daily Express*, 8 February, 25.
32. Tan, S.I. & Jacobs, H.S. (1991). *Infertility: Your Questions Answered.* London: McGraw Hill.
33. Pfeffer, N. & Woollett, A. (1983). *The Experience of Infertility.* London: Virago.
34. Editional, (1993). Too old to have a baby. *Lancet, 341*, 344–5.
35. Jardine, C. (1993). I had a baby at 55. *Woman*, 30 August.
36. Bennion, F. (1987). Letter entitled 'New age for birth' *Independent*, 14 September.
37. Narayan, H., Buckett, W., McDougall, W. & Cullimore, J. (1992). Pregnancy after fifty: profile and pregnancy outcome in a series of elderly multigravidae. *European Journal of Obstetrics, Gynecology & Reproductive Biology, 47* (1), 47–51.
38. Matthew, P. (ed) (1994). *The Guinness Book of Records.* Section on Reproductivity. London: Guinness Publishing (see page 62).
39. Sauer, M.V., Paulson, R.J. & Lobo, R.A. (1993). Pregnancy after age 50: application of oocyte donation for women after natural menopause. *Lancet, 341*, 321–3.
40. Phillip, J. (1994). Woman, 62, gives birth as 'oldest mother in world'. *The Times*, 19 July.
41. Lawrence, C. (1991). Making age a thing of the past. *Daily Telegraph*, 29 October.

3: Why have Babies after 35? Decision-Making and Later Parenthood

1. Freely, M. & Pyper, C. (1993). *Pandora's Clock: Understanding our Fertility.* London: Heinemann.
2. Wallach, H.R. & Maitlin, M.W. (1992). College women's expectations about pregnancy, childbirth and infant care: A prospective study. *Birth, 19*, 202–207.
3. Griffin, C. (1985). *Typical Girls: Young Women from School to the Job-Market.* London: Routledge.
4. Lees, S. (1986). *Losing Out: Sexuality and Adolescent Girls.* London: Hutchinson.
5. Woollett, A. (1991). Having Children: Accounts of childless women and women with reproductive problems. In A. Phoenix, A. Woollett & E. Lloyd (eds) *Motherhood: Meanings, Practices and Ideologies.* London: Sage.
6. Donnis, S. (1984). Common themes of infertility: a counselling

model. *Journal of Sex Education and Therapy*, *10*, 11–15.

7. Berryman, J.C. (1993). Who wants egg donation? *Issue*, Winter, 13–14.

8. Soloway, N.M. & Smith, R.M. (1987). Antecedents of late-timing birth decisions of men and women in dual-career marriages. *Family Relations*, *36*, 258–62.

9. Thorpe, K.J. & Cinnamon, J. (1992). The Timing of Motherhood. Unpublished research report. University of Queensland. Australia.

10. Oakley, A. (1981). *From Here to Maternity: Becoming a Mother*. London: Penguin.

11. Monarch, J. (1991). *Childless-no-Choice*. London: Routledge.

12. Cooper, C. & Davidson, M. (1982). *High Pressure: Working Lives of Women Managers*. London: Fontana.

13. Hoffman, L.W. & Nye, F.I. (1975). *Working Mothers*. San Francisco: Jossey-Bass.

14. Roland, A. & Harris, B. (1979). *Career and Motherhood*. New York: Human Sciences Press.

15. Troll, L.E. (1985). *Early and Middle Adulthood* (2nd edition). Monterey, CA: Brooks Cole.

16. Brannen, J. & Moss, P. (1988). *New Mothers at Work*. London: Unwin.

17. Nicholson, N. & West, M.A. (1988). *Managerial Job Change: Men and Women in Transition*. Cambridge University Press.

18. Cohen, B. (1988). *Caring for Children: Services and Policies for Childcare and Equal Opportunities in the United Kingdom. Report for the European Commissions Childcare Network*. London: Family Policy Studies Centre.

19. Bram, S. (19178). Through the looking glass: Voluntary childlessness as a mirror to contemporary changes in the meaning of parenthood. In W.B. Miller & L. Newman (eds) *The First Child and Family Formation*. Chapel Hill: North Carolina Population Centre.

20. Shultz, T. (1979). *Women Can Wait: The Measures of Motherhood after Thirty*. New York: Doubleday.

21. National Childbirth Trust. (1994). Is there sex after childbirth? *New Generation*, *13*, 24–5.

22. Thorpe, K.J., Dragonas, T. & Golding, J. (1992). The effects of psychosocial factors on the mother's emotional well-being during early parenthood: a cross-cultural study of Britain and Greece. *Journal of Reproductive and Infant Psychology*, *10*, 191–204.

23. Stewart, D.E. & Robinson, G.E. (1989). Infertility by choice or by nature. *Canadian Journal of Psychiatry*, *34*, 866–71.

24. Veevers, J. (1980). *Childless by Choice*. Toronto: Butterworths.

25. Johnson, G. (1993). Childless women revisited. *British Medical Journal*, *307*, 1116–7.

26. Callan, V.J. (1986). Pregnancy as seen by mothers wanting one or

two children, voluntarily childless wives and single women. *Australian Journal of Sex, Marriage and the Family*, 7(2), 83–9.

27. Callan, V.J. (1986). The impact of the first birth: married and single women preferring childlessness, one child and two children. *Journal of Marriage and the Family*, 48, 261–9.

28. Reading, J. & Amatea, E.S. (1986). Role deviance or role diversification: Reassessing the psycho-social factors affecting the parenthood choice of career orientated women. *Journal of Marriage and the Family*, 48, 255–60.

29. Daniluk, J.C. & Herman, A.L. (1984). Parenthood decision-making. *Family Relations*, 33, 607–12.

30. Michaels, G.Y. (1988). Motivational factors in the decision and timing of pregnancy. in G.Y. Michaels & W.A. Goldberg (eds) *Transition to Parenthood: Current Theory and Research*. Cambridge University Press.

31. Guillebaud, J. (1985). *Contraception: your questions answered*. London: Pitman.

32. Ory, H.W. (1983). Mortality associated with fertility and fertility control. *Family Planning Perspectives*, 15, 57–63.

33. Lester, C. & Farrow, S. (1988). Unwanted pregnancies at ante-natal clinic. *Midwifery*, 4, 184–9.

34. MacIntyre, S. (1976). To have or not to have – promotion and prevention of childbirth in gynaecological work. In M. Stacey (ed) *The Sociology of the NHS*. University of Keele, UK.

35. While. A.E. (1990). The incidence of unplanned and unwanted pregnancies among live births from health visitor records. *Child: Care Health and Development*, 16, 219–26.

36. Avon Longitudinal Study of Pregnancy and Childhood (ALSPAC). Unpublished figures with the kind permission of Professor Jean Golding, Institute of Child Health, University of Bristol, UK.

37. Berryman, J.C. & Windridge, K.C. (1991). Having a baby after 40: A preliminary investigation of women's experience of pregnancy. *Journal of Reproductive and Infant Psychology*, 9, 3–18.

38. Berryman, J.C. (1991). Perspectives on later motherhood. In A. Phoenix, A. Woollett & E. Lloyd (eds) *Motherhood: Meanings, Practices and Ideologies*. London: Sage.

39. Central Statistics Office. (1989). *General Household Survey, 1986: An Inter-departmental survey*. London: HMSO.

40. Desper, B. (1992). When to have a baby: An obstetrical point of view. *Journal of the American Medical Women's Association*, 47, 75–6.

41. Schlesinger, B. & Schlesinger, R. (1989). Postponed parenthood: trends and issues. *Journal of Comparative Family Studies*, 20, 355–63.

42. Presser, H. (1978). In W.B. Miller & L. Newman (eds) *The First Child and Family Formation*. Chapel Hill: North Carolina Population Centre.

43. Kalache, Amaguire, A. & Thomson, S.G. (1993). Age at last full-term pregnancy and risk of breast cancer. *Lancet, 341*, 33–6.

44. Kvale, G., Heuch, I. & Nilssen, S. (1992). Endometrial cancer and age at last delivery: evidence for an association. *American Journal of Epidemiology, 135* (4), 453–5.

45. Cummings, P., Stanford, J.L., Daling, J.R., Weiss, N.S. & McKnight, B. (1994). Risk of breast cancer in relation to the interval since last full-term pregnancy. *British Medical Journal, 308* 1672–2674.

46. Berryman, J.C. & Windridge, K.C. (1994). Leicester Motherhood Project. Unpublished figures. University of Leicester, UK.

47. Bryan, E., Higgins, R. & Harvey, D. (1991). Ethical issues. In D. Harvey & E. Bryan (eds) *The Stress of Multiple Birth*. Queen Charlotte's and Chelsea Hospital, London: Multiple Births Foundation.

48. Collee, J. (1991). A doctor writes: Anna's choice. *Observer* Magazine.

49. Thorpe, K.J., Golding, J., Greenwood, R. & MacGillivray, I. (1991). A comparison of the prevalence of depression in the mothers of twins and the mothers of singletons. *British Medical Journal, 302*, 875–8.

50. James, D.K. (1988). Risk at the booking clinic. In D.K. James and G.M. Stirratt (eds) *Pregnancy and Risk: The basis for rational management*. Chicester: John Wiley and Sons.

51. Lamb, J. (1993). Four Ages of Motherhood, *Mother and Baby*.

52. Hoffman, L.W. (1977). Changes in family roles, socialisation and sex differences. *American Psychologist, 32*, 644–58.

53. Daniels, P. & Weingarten, K. (1982). *Sooner or Later: The Timing of Parenthood in Adult Lives*. New York: W.W. Norton.

4: 'Trying' for a Baby after 35: Getting and Staying Pregnant

1. Brew, J. Cited in I. Kern, (1982). '. . . an endless joy . . .': The culture of motherhood over 35. *Papers in the Social Sciences, 2*, 43–56.

2. Gindoff, P.R. & Jewelewicz, R. (1986). Reproductive potential in the older woman. *Fertility & Sterility, 46* (6), 989–1001.

3. Bourne, G. (1989). *Pregnancy*. London: Pan Books.

4. Eaton, J.W. & Mayer, A.J. (1953). The social biology of very high fertility among the Hutterites: The demography of a unique population. *Human Biology, 25* (3), 206–64.

5. Tietze, C. (1957). Reproductive span and rate of reproduction among Hutterite women. *Fertility and Sterility, 8* (1), 89–97.

6. Henry, L. (1961). Some data on natural fertility. *Eugenics Quarterly, 8*, 81–91.

7. Schwartz, D. & Mayaux, M.J. (1982). Female fecundity as a function of age. *New England Journal of Medicine, 306* (7), 404–6.
8. Mosher, W.D. (1982). Infertility trends among U.S. couples: 1965–1976. *Family Planning Perspectives. 14* (22), 22–7.
9. Gosden, R.G. (1985). *Biology of Menopause: The Causes and Consequences of Ovarian Ageing.* London: Academic Press (see page 95).
10. Berryman, J.C. & Windridge, K.C. (1994). Leicester Motherhood Project. Unpublished findings. University of Leicester, UK.
11. Berryman, J.C. & Windridge, K.C. (1991). Having a baby after 40: I. A preliminary investigation of women's experience of pregnancy. *Journal of Reproductive and Infant Psychology, 9,* 3–18.
12. *General Household Survey, 1986.* (1989). An Inter-departmental survey sponsored by the Central Statistical Office. London: HMSO.
13. Cartwright, A. (1976). *How Many Children?* London: Routledge and Kegan Paul.
14. Short, R.V. (1976). The evolution of human reproduction. *Proceedings of the Royal Society of London, 195,* 3–24 (see page 493).
15. Katchadourian, H. (1977). Cited in Coleman, J.C. (1980). *The Nature of Adolescence.* London: Methuen.
16. Zaadstra, B.M., Seidell, J.C., Van Noord., te Velde E.R., Habbema J.D.F., Vrieswijk, B. & Karbaat, J. (1993). Fat and female fecundity: prospective study of effect of body fat distribution on conception rates. *British Medical Journal, 306,* 484–7.
17. May, R.M. (1978). Human reproduction reconsidered. *Nature, 272,* 491–5.
18. Gellen, J.J. (1992). The feasibility of suppressing ovarian activity following the end of amenorrhoea by increasing the frequency of sucking. *International Journal of Gynaecology & Obstetrics, 39* (4), 321–5.
19. Kitzinger, S. (1982). *Birth Over Thirty.* London: Sheldon Press.
20. Suonio, S., Saarikoski, O., Kauhanen, O., Metsäpelto, A., Terho, J. & Vohlonen, I. (1990). Smoking does affect fecundity. *European Journal of Obstetrics & Gynecology and Reproductive Biology, 34,* 89–95.
21. Baird, D.D. & Wilcox, A.J. (1985). Cigarette smoking associated with delayed conception. *Journal of the American Medical Association, 253,* 2979–83.
22. Wilcox, A., Weinberg, C. & Baird, D. (1988). Caffeinated beverages and decreased fertility. *Lancet, 2,* 1453–5.
23. Grodstein, F., Goldman, M.B., Ryan, L. & Cramer, D.W. (1993). Relation of female infertility to consumption of caffeinated beverages. *American Journal of Epidemiology, 137* (12), 1353–60.
24. Tan, S.I. & Jacobs, H.S. (1992). *Infertility: Your Questions Answered.* London: McGraw Hill.

25. Redgment, C.J., Al-Shawaf, T., Grudzinskas, J.G. & Craft, I.L. (1994). Gamete intrafallopian transfer in older women: effect of limiting number of gametes transferred. *British Medical Journal*, *309*, 510–11.
26. Freely, M. & Pyper, C. (1993). *Pandora's Clock: Understanding our Fertility*. London: Heinemann.
27. Abdalla, H.I., Burton, G., Kirkland, A., Johnson, M.R., Leonard, T., Brooks, A.A. & Studd, J.W.W. (1993). Age, pregnancy and miscarriage: uterine versus ovarian factors. *Human Reproduction, 8* (9), 1512–1517.
28. Rogers, L. (1994). Ovary donor cards urged for all women. *The Times*, 19 June.
29. Gosden, R.G. (1992). Transplantation of fetal germ cells. *Journal of Assisted Reproduction & Genetics, 9* (2), 118–23.
30. Sauer, M.V., Paulson, R.J. & Lobo, R.A. (1992). Reversing the natural decline in human fertility. An extended clinical trial of oocyte donation to women of advanced reproductive age. *Journal of the American Medical Association. 9*:268 (10), 1275–9.
31. Antinori, S. Cited in J. Phillips (1994). Woman, 62 gives birth as 'oldest mother in the world'. *The Times*, 19 July.
32. Winston, R. Cited in Freely, M. & Pyper, C. (1993). *Pandora's Clock: Understanding Our Fertility*. London: Heinemann (see page 228).
33. Warnock, M. cited in A. Neustatter (1993). Pioneer in the laboratory of life. *Independent*, 3 August.
34. *Birth Statistics, 1992*. (1994). Review of the Registrar General on births and patterns of family building in England and Wales. Series FM1. no 21. London: HMSO.
35. Gilot, F. & Lake, C. (1964). *Life with Picasso*. London: Penguin.
36. Craft, I. Cited in A. Neustatter (1993). Pioneer in the laboratory of life. *Independent*, 3 August.
37. Simpson, J.L. (1990). Incidence and timing of pregnancy losses: relevance to evaluating safety of early prenatal diagnosis. *American Journal of Medical Genetics, 35*, 165–73.
38. Warburton, D. & Fraser, F.C. (1964). Spontaneous abortion risks in man. Data from reproductive histories collected in a medical genetics units. *American Journal of Human Genetics, 16*, 1–25.
39. Hansen, J. (1986). Older maternal age and pregnancy outcome: a review of the literature. *Obstetrical & Gynecological Survey, 41* (11), 726–34.
40. Llewellyn-Jones, D. (1982). *Everywoman: A Gynaecological Guide for Life*. London: Faber & Faber.
41. Virro M.R. & Shewchuk, A.B. (1984). Pregnancy outcome in 242 conceptions after artificial insemination with donor sperm and effects of maternal age on the prognosis for successful pregnancy. *American Journal of Obstetrics and Gynecology, 148*, 518–24.

5: What are the Risks? The Evidence on Problems associated with Later Motherhood

1. Collee, J. (1991). A doctor writes. *Observer* Magazine.
2. James, D.K. (1988). Risk at the booking visit. In D.K. James & G.M. Stirratt (eds) *Pregnancy and Risk: The Rational Basis for Management*. Chicester: John Wiley and Sons.
3. Donnai, D. (1988). Genetic risk. In D.K. James & G.M. Stirratt (eds) *Pregnancy and Risk: The Rational Basis for Management*. Chichester: John Wiley and Sons.
4. Finch, C.E. and Gosden, R.G. (1984). Animal Models for the Human Menopause. In L. Mastroianni & C.A. Paulsen (eds) *Aging, Reproduction and the Climacteric*. New York: Plenum.
5. Jongbloet, P.H. (1986). Prepregnancy care: Background biological effects. In G. Chamberlain & J. Lumley, *Prepregnancy Care: a Manual for Practice*. London: John Wiley and Sons.
6. Hook, E.B. (1981). Rates of chromosomal abnormality at different maternal ages. *Obstetrics and Gynaecology*, *58*, 282–5.
7. MacGillivray, I. (1988). Management of twin pregnancy. In I. MacGillivray, D.M. Campbell & B. Thompson (eds) *Twins and Twinning*. Chichester: John Wiley and Sons.
8. Cooke, R. (1991). Neonatal problems. In D. Harvey & E. Bryan. *The Stress of Multiple Birth*. Queen Charlotte's and Chelsea Hospital, London: Multiple Birth Foundation.
9. Hansen, J. (1986). Older maternal age and pregnancy outcome: a review of the literature. *Obstetrics and Gynaecology*, *41* (11), 726–34.
10. Warbuton, D. & Fraser, F.C. (1964). Spontaneous abortion risks in man. Data from reproductive histories collected in a medical genetics unit. *American Journal of Human Genetics*, *16*, 1–25.
11. Stoppard, M. (1993). *Pregnancy, Conception and Birth*. London: Dorling Kindersley.
12. MacDonald, I.R. & Maclennon, H.R. (1960). A consideration of the treatment of the elderly primigravidae. *Journal of Obstetrics and Gynaecology of the British Empire*, *67*, 443–50.
13. Grimes, D.A. & Gross, G.K. (1981). Pregnancy outcomes in black women aged 35 and older. *Obstetrics and Gynaecology*, *52*, 7–12.
14. Kessler, I., Lancet, M., Borenstein, R. & Steinmetz, A. (1980). The problem of the elderly primigravida. *Obstetrics and Gynaecology*, *56*. 165–9.
15. Messinis, I., Malamitsi-Puchner, A. & Hadjigeorgiou, E. (1982) Cited by R. Resnick, Pregnancy in women aged 35 years and older In D.R. Hollingsworth, and R. Resnick (eds) *Medical Counselling Before Pregnancy*. New York: Churchill Livingstone.
16. Caspi, E. & Lifshitz, Y. (1979). Delivery at 40 years of age and over

Israeli Journal of Medical Science, 15, 418–21.

17. Kajunsuu, P., Kivinen, S. & Tuimala, R. (1981). Pregnancy and delivery at the age of forty and over. *International Journal of Obstetrics and Gynaecology, 19,* 341–5.

18. Horger, E.O. & Smythe, A.R. (1977). Pregnancy in women over 40. *Obstetrics and Gynaecology, 49,* 257–60.

19. Spellacy, W.N., Miller, S.J. & Winegar, A. (1986). Pregnancy after 40 years of age. *Obstetrics and Gynaecology, 68,* 452–4.

20. Kirz, D.S., Dorchester, W. & Freeman, R.K. (1985). Advanced maternal age: the mature primigravida. *American Journal of Obstetrics and Gynaecology, 152,* 7–12.

21. Berkowitz, G.S., Skovron, M.L., Lapinski, R.H. & Berkowitz, R.L. (1990). Delayed childbearing and the outcome of pregnancy. *New England Journal of Medicine, 10:322,* 659–64.

22. Piepert, J.F. & Bracken, M.B. (1993). Maternal age: An independent risk factor for cesarean section. *Obstetrics and Gynaecology, 81,* 200–205.

23. Stanton, E. (1956). Pregnancy after forty-four. *American Journal of Obstetrics and Gynaecology, 71,* 270–84.

24. Friedman, E. (1965). Relation of maternal age to the course of labor. *American Journal of Obstetrics and Gynaecology, 91,* 915–23.

25. Morrison, I. (1975). The elderly primigravida. *American Journal of Obstetrics and Gynaecology, 121,* 465–70.

26. Cohen, W.R., Newman, L. & Friedman, E.A. (1980). Risk of labor abnormalities with advancing maternal age. *Obstetrics and Gynaecology, 55,* 414–16.

27. Stein, A. (1983). Pregnancy in gravidas over age 35 years. *Nurse Midwife, 28* (1), 17–20.

28. Biggs, J.S.G. (1973). Pregnancy at 40 years and over. *Medical Journal of Australia, 1,* 542.

29. Koren, Z. (1963). Pregnancy and birth over 40. *Obstetrics and Gynaecology, 21,* 165–9.

30. Horger, E. & Smythe, A.R. (1977). Pregnancy in women over 40. *Obstetrics and Gynaecology, 49,* 257–61.

31. Israel, S.L. & Deutschberger, J. (1964). Relation of the mother's age to obstetric performance. *Obstetrics and Gynaecology, 24,* 411–17.

32. Berryman, J.C. & Windridge, K.C. (1994). Leicester Motherhood Project. Unpublished findings. University of Leicester, UK.

33. Mor-yosef, S., Samueloff, A., Moden, B., Navot, D. & Scenker, J.G. (1990). Ranking the risk factors for cesarean: logistic regression analysis of a nation wide study. *Obstetrics and Gynaecology, 75,* 944–7.

34. Kane, S. (1967). Advancing age and the primigravida. *Obstetrics and Gynaecology, 29,* 409–14.

35. Department of Health. (1991). Report of the Confidential Enquiry

into Maternal Deaths in the United Kingdom, 1985–7. London: HMSO.

36. MacMahon, B., Cole. P. & Brown, J. (1973). Etiology of human breast cancer: a review. *Journal of National Cancer Institute, 50,* 21–42.

37. Kelsey, J.L. & Hildreth, N.G. (1983). *Breast and gynecologic cancer epidemiology.* Boca Raton, Florida: CRC Press.

38. Logan, W.P.D. (1953). Marriage and childbearing in relation to cancer of the breast and uterus. *Lancet, ii,* 1199–202.

39. Hseih, C., Goldman, M., Pavia, M., Ekbom, A., Peridou, E., Adami, H-O. & Trichopoulos, D. (1993). Breast cancer risks in mothers of multiple births, *International Journal of Cancer, 54,* 81–4.

40. Cummings, P., Stanford, J.L., Daling, J.L., Weiss, N.S. & McKnight, B. (1994). Risk of breast cancer in relation to the interval since last full-term pregnancy. *British Medical Journal, 308,* 1672–4.

41. Bruzzi, P., Negri, E., La Vecchia, C., Decarli, A., Palli, D. & Parrazinni, F. (1988). Short term increase in risk of breast cancer after full-term pregnancy. *British Medical Journal, 297,* 1096–8.

42. Williams, E.M.I., Jones, L., Vessey, M.P. & McPherson, K. (1990). Short term increase in the risk of breast cancer following full-term pregnancy. *British Medical Journal, 300,* 578–9.

43. Adami, H., Bergstom, R., Lund, E., & Meirik, O. (1990). Absence of association between reproductive variables and risk of breast cancer in young women in Sweden and Norway. *British Journal of Cancer, 62,* 122–6.

44. Vatten, L.J. & Kvinnsland, S. (1992). Pregnancy related factors and risk of breast cancer in a prospective study of 29,981 Norwegian women. *European Journal of Cancer, 28A,* 1148–53.

45. MacMahon, B., Cole, P., Lin, T.M., Lowe, C.R., Mirra, A.P. & Ravinhar, B. (1970). Age at first birth and breast cancer risk. *Bulletin of the WHO, 42,* 209–21.

46. Kalache, A., Maguire, A. & Thompson, S.G. (1993). Age at last full-term pregnancy and risk of breast cancer. *Lancet, 341,* 33–6.

47. Miller, A. (1984). Cancer of the breast. In K. Magnus (ed) *Trends in cancer incidence.* New York: Hemisphere Publishing.

48. Lesko, S.M., Rosenberg, L. & Kaufman, D.W. (1991). Endometrial cancer and age at last delivery: evidence for an association. *American Journal of Epidemiology, 133,* 554–9.

49. Kvale, G., Heuch, I. & Nilssen, S. (1992). Endometrial cancer and age at last delivery: evidence for an association. *American Journal of Epidemiology, 135,* (4), 453–5.

50. Kvale, G., Heuch, I. & Ursin, G. (1988). Reproductive factors and risk of breast cancer of the uterine corpus: a prospective study. *Cancer Research, 48,* 6217–21.

51. Bakkerteig, L. & Hoffman, H.J. (1981). Epidemiology of pre-term birth: results from a longitudinal study of births in Norway. In Elder, M.G. & Hofman, H.J. (eds) *Obstetrics and Gynaecology I: Preterm Labour.* London: Butterworths (pp. 17–46).

52. Forman, M.R., Meirik, O. & Berendes, H.W. (1984). Delayed childbearing in Sweden. *Journal of the American Medical Association,* 252, 3135–9.

53. Keily, J.L., Paneth, N. & Susser, M. (1986). An assessment of the effects of maternal age and parity in different components of perinatal mortality. *American Journal of Epidemiology, 123,* 444–54.

54. Barken, S.E. & Bracken, M.B. (1987). Delayed childbearing: No evidence for increased risk of low birthweight and pre-term delivery. *American Journal of Epidemiology, 125,* 101–9.

55. Welles-Nystrom, B.L. & de Chateau, P. (1987). Maternal age and transition to motherhood: prenatal and perinatal assessment. *Acta Psychiatrica Scandinavica, 76,* 719–25.

56. Baird, P.A., Sadovnick, A.D. & Yee, I.M.L. (1991). Maternal age and birth defects: a population study. *Lancet, 337,* 527–30.

57. Dalen, P. (1977). Maternal age and the incidence of schizophrenia in the Republic of Ireland. *British Journal of Psychiatry, 131,* 301–5.

58. Gardener, M.J., Snee, M.P., Hall, A.J., Powell, C.A., Downes, S. & Terrell, J.D. (1990). Results of case control study of leukemia and lymphoma near Sellafield nuclear plant in West Cumbria. *British Medical Journal, 300,* 423–34.

59. Berryman, J.C. (1991). Perspectives on later motherhood. In A Phoenix, A. Woollett and E. Lloyd (eds) *Motherhood: Meanings, Practices and Ideologies.* London: Sage.

60. Mansfield, P.K. (1988). Midlife childbearing: strategies for informed decisionmaking. *Psychology of Women Quarterly, 12,* 445–60.

61. Whittle, M.J. (1993). Screening for Down's Syndrome. *British Journal of Midwifery, 1* (3), 109.

62. Katz Rothman, B. (1986). *The Tentative Pregnancy.* New York: Viking Penguin.

63. Barbour, R.S. (1990). Fathers: the emergence of a new consumer group. In J. Garcia, R. Kilpatrick and M.P.M. Richards (eds) *The Politics of Maternity Care.* Oxford University Press.

64. Mansfield, P.K. & Cohn, M.D. (1986). Stress and later life childbearing: important implications for nursing. *Maternal Child Nursing Journal, 15,* 139–51.

65. Reid, M. (1990). Prenatal diagnosis and screening. In J. Garcia, R. Kilpatrick and M.P.M. Richards (eds) *The Politics of Maternity Care.* Oxford University Press.

66. Richards, M.P.M. (1989). Social and ethical problems of fetal diagnosis and screening. *Journal of Reproductive and Infant Psychology, 7,* 171–86.

67. Kitzinger, S. (1982). *Birth Over Thirty*, London: Sheldon Press.

6: Pregnancy after 35: The Experience

1. Berryman, J.C. & Windridge, K.C. (1991). Having a baby after 40: I. A preliminary investigation of women's experience of pregnancy. *Journal of Reproductive and Infant Psychology, 9*, 3–18.
2. Berryman, J.C. & Windridge, K.C. Leicester Motherhood Project. (1994). Unpublished findings. University of Leicester, UK.
3. Green, J. Statham, H. & Snowdon, C. (1993). Women's knowledge of prenatal screening tests. I: Relationship with hospital screening policy and demographic factors. *Journal of Reproductive and Infant Psychology, 11*, 11–20.
4. Marteau, T., Johnson, M., Plenicar, M., Shaw, R. & Slack, J. (1988). Development of a self-administered questionnaire to measure women's knowledge of prenatal screening and diagnostic tests. *Journal of Psychosomatic Research, 32*, 403–8.
5. Evans, M., Pryde, P., Evans, W. & Johnson, M. (1993). The choices women make about prenatal diagnosis. *Fetal Diagnosis and Therapy, 8*, 70–80.
6. Roelofsen, E., Kamerbeek, L. & Tymstra, Tj. (1993). Chances and Choices: Psychosocial consequences of maternal serum screening. A report from the Netherlands. *Journal of Reproductive and Infant Psychology, 11*, 41–7. See pp. 43 and 44.
7. Rapp, R. (1987). Moral pioneers: women, men and fetuses on a frontier of reproductive technology. *Women and Health, 13* (1–2), 101–16. Quote from p.113.
8. Green, J.M. (1990). Calming or Harming? A critical review of psychological effects of fetal diagnosis on pregnant women. *Galton Institute Occasional Paper*, Second Series, No.2.
9. Wertz, D. (1993). Providers' gender and moral reasoning: A proposed agenda for research on providers and patients. *Fetal Diagnosis and Therapy, 8*, 81–9. Quote from p.81.
10. Marteau, T., Plenicar, M. & Kidd, J. (1993). Obstetricians presenting amniocentesis to pregnant women: practice observed. *Journal of Reproductive and Infant Psychology, 11*, 3–10.
11. Marteau, T. (1989). The ethics of clinical research. *British Medical Journal, 299*, 513–14.
12. Ley, P. (1988). *Communicating with Patients: Improving Communication, Satisfaction, and Compliance*. London: Croom-Helm.
13. Harper, P. (1991). *Practical Genetic Counselling, 3rd edition*. Oxford: Butterworth-Heinemann.
14. Marteau, T. (1989). Framing of information: its influence upon

decisions of doctors and patients. *British Journal of Social Psychology*, *28*, 89–94.

15. Van Zuuren, F. (1993). Coping style and anxiety during prenatal diagnosis. *Journal of Reproductive and Infant Psychology*, *11*, 57–9.

16. Khalid, L., Price, S. & Barrow, M. (1994). The attitude of midwives to maternal serum screening for Down's syndrome. *Public Health*, *108*, 131–6.

17. Welles-Nystrom, B.L. & de Chateau, P. (1987). Maternal age and transition to parenthood: prenatal and perinatal assessment. *Acta Psychiatrica Scandinavica*, *76*, 719–25.

18. Fava, G.A., Grandi, S., Michelacci, L., Saviotti, F., Conti, S., Bovicelli, L., Trombini, G. & Orlandi, C. (1990). Hypochondriacal fears and beliefs in pregnancy. *Acta Psychiatrica Scandinavica*, *82*, 70–2.

19. Pagel, M.D., Smilkstein, G., Regen, H. & Montano, D. (1990). Psychosocial influences on new born outcomes: a controlled prospective study. *Social Science and Medicine*, *30* (5), 597–604.

20. Van den Burgh, B.R. (1990). The influence of maternal emotions during pregnancy on fetal and neonatal behaviour. *Pre and Perinatal Psychology Journal*, *5* (2), 119–30.

21. Field, T., Sandberg, D., Quetel, T., Garcia, R., Rosario, M. (1985). Effects of ultrasound feedback on pregnancy anxiety, fetal activity and neonatal outcome. *Obstetrics and Gynecology*, *66*, 525–8.

22. Zeanah, C.H., Carr, S. & Wolk, S. (1990). Fetal movements and the imagined baby of pregnancy: are they related? *Journal of Reproductive and Infant Psychology*, *8*, 23–36.

23. Lewis, J. (1988). The transition to parenthood: II. Stability and change in marital structure. *Family Process*, *27*, 273–83.

24. Jones, K. (1990). Expectant Fears. *Nursing Times*, *86* (15), 36–8.

25. Harker, L. & Thorpe, K. (1992). 'The last egg in the basket?' Elderly primiparity–A review of findings. *Birth*, *19:1*, 23–30.

26. Thorpe, K.J., Greenwood, R. & Little, R.E. (1994). Frequency of alcohol use, life events, and emotional status in pregnancy. University of Bristol, UK: Manuscript submitted for publication.

27. Children of the Nineties: data from the Avon Longitudinal Study of Pregnancy and Childhood. Supplied by Greenwood, R. with permission of Golding, J.University of Bristol, UK.

28. Robinson, G.E., Garner, D.M., Gare, D.J. & Crawford, B. (1987). Psychological adaptation to pregnancy in childless women more than 35 years of age. *American Journal of Obstetrics and Gynecology*, *156* (2), 328–33.

29. Fleming, A.S., Flett, G.L., Ruble, D.N. & Van Wagner, V. (1990). Adjustment in first-time mothers: changes in mood content during the early postpartum months. *Developmental Psychology*, *26* (1), 137–43.

30. Green, J.M. (1990). 'Who is Unhappy after Childbirth?' Antenatal and intrapartum correlates from a prospective study. *Journal of Reproductive and Infant Psychology, 8* (3), 175–83.

31. Oates, M. (1989). Normal emotional changes in pregnancy and the puerperium. *Baillieres Clinical Obstetrics and Gynaecology, 3* (4), 791–804.

32. Robinson, G.E., Olmsted, M., Garner, D.M. & Gare, D.J. (1988). Transition to parenthood in elderly primiparas. *Journal of Psychosomatic Obstetrics and Gynaecology, 9*, 89–101.

33. Mercer, R. (1986). *First Time Motherhood. Experiences from Teens to Forties.* New York: Springer.

34. Gottesman, M.M. (1992). Maternal adaptation during pregnancy among adult early, middle, and late childbearers: Similarities and Differences. *Maternal-Child Nursing Journal, 20* (2), 93–110.

35. Jarrahi-Zadeh, A., Kane, F.J. Jr., Van De Castle, R.L., Lachenbruch, P.A. & Ewing, J.A. (1969). Emotional and cognitive changes in pregnancy and early puerperium. *British Journal of Psychiatry, 115* (3), 797–805.

36. Groner, J.A., Holtzman, N.A., Charney, E. & Mellits, E. (1986). A randomised trial or oral iron on tests of short-term memory and attention span in young pregnant women. *Journal of Adolescent Health Care, 7* (1), 44–8.

37. Parsons, C. and Redman, S. (1991). Self-reported cognitive change during pregnancy. *The Australian Journal of Advanced Nursing, 9* (1), 20–9.

38. Wellings, K., Field, J., Johnson, A & Wadsworth, J. (1994). *Sexual Behaviour in Britain. The National Survey of Sexual Attitudes and Lifestyles.* London: Penguin.

39. Kinsey, A., Pomeroy, W., Martin, C. & Gebhard, P. (1953). *Sexual Behaviour in the Human Female.* W.B. Saunders, Philadelphia.

40. Reamy, K. & White, S. (1985). Sexuality in pregnancy and the puerperium: a review. *Obstetrical and Gynecological Survey, 40* (1), 1–13 (see page 4).

41. Bailey, v. (1989). Sexuality – before and after birth. *Midwives Chronicle and Nursing Notes, 102* (1212), 24–6.

42. Walbroehl, G.S. (1984). Sexuality during pregnancy. *American Family Physician, 29* (5), 273–5.

43. Aaronson, L.S. (1989). Perceived and received support: effects on health behaviour during pregnancy. *Nursing Research, 38* (1), 4–9.

44. Devoe, L.D., Murray, C., Youssif, A & Arnaud, M. (1993). Maternal caffeine consumption and fetal behaviour in normal third-trimester pregnancy. *American Journal of Obstetrics and Gynecology, 168* (4), 1105–11.

45. Seidman, D.S., Ever-Hadani, P. & Gale, R. (1990). Effect of maternal smoking and age on congenital anomalies. *Obstetrics and*

Gynecology, *76* (6), 1046–50.
46. Kandel, D.B. (1990). Parenting styles, drug use, and children's adjustment in families of young adults. *Journal of Marriage and the Family*, *52*, 183–96.
47. Ostrea, E.M., Brady, M., Raymundo, A.L. & Stevens, M. (1992). Drug screening of newborns by meconium analysis: a large-scale, prospective, epidemiologic study. *Pediatrics*, *89* (1), 107–13.
48. Tinsley, B.J., Trupin, S.R., Owens, L. & Boyum, LA. (1993). The significance of women's pregnancy-related locus of control beliefs for adherence to recommended prenatal health regimens and pregnancy outcomes. *Journal of Reproductive and Infant Psychology*, *11*, 97–102.
49. Bielawska-Batorowicz, E. (1993). The effect of previous obstetric history on women's scores on the Fetal Health Locus of Control Scale (FHLC). *Journal of Reproductive and Infant Psychology*, *11*, 103–6.
50. Muller, M.E. (1993). Development of the prenatal attachment inventory. *Western Journal of Nursing Research*, *15* (2), 199–215.
51. Berryman, J.C. & Windridge, K.C. (1993). Pregnancy after 35: a preliminary report on maternal-fetal attachment. *Journal of Reproductive and Infant Psychology*, *11*, 169–74.
52. Statham, H. & Green, J. (1993). Serum screening for Down's syndrome: some women's experiences. *British Medical Journal*, *307*, 174–6.

7: Self and Others: the Mother's Social World

1. Winnubst, J., Buunk, B., & Marcelissen, F. (1988). Social support and stress: Perspectives and processes. In S. Fisher & J. Reason (eds) *Handbook of Life Stress, Cognition and Health*. Chichester: John Wiley and Sons.
2. Younger, J.B. (1991). A model of parenting stress. *Research in Nursing and Health*, *14* (3), 197–204.
3. Headey, B. & Wearing, A. (1989). Personality, life events, and subjective well-being: toward a dynamic equilibrium model. *Journal of Personality and Social Psychology*, *57* (4), 731–9.
4. Fleetwood Mac, *Rumours*.
5. Rossan, S. (1994). Personal communication with J.C. Berryman, University of Leicester, UK.
6. Gilligan, C. (1982). *In a Different Voice: Psychological Theory and Women's Development*. Cambridge, Massachusetts: Harvard University Press (see page 17).
7. Guttman, D. (1977). The cross-cultural perspective: notes towards

a comparative psychology of ageing. In J.E. Birren & K.W. Schaie (eds) *Handbook of the Psychology of Ageing*. New York: Van Nostrand Reinhold.

8. Kern, I. (1982). '. . . an endless joy . . .': The culture of motherhood over 35. *Papers in the Social Sciences*, *2*, 43–56 (see pages 54 and 50).

9. Berryman, J.C. & Windridge, K.C. (1994). Leicester Motherhood Project. Unpublished findings. University of Leicester, UK.

10. Robinson, G.E., Olmsted, M., Garner, D.M. & Gare, D.J. (1988). Transition to parenthood in elderly primiparas. *Journal of Psychosomatic Obstetrics and Gynaecology*, *9*, 89–101.

11. Helson, R., Mitchell, V. & Moane, G. (1984). Personality and patterns of adherence and nonadherence to the social clock. *Journal of Personality and Social Psychology*, *46* (5), 1079–96.

12. *Birth Statistics, 1987*. (1989). Review of the Registrar General on births and patterns of family building in England and Wales. Series FM1, no. 16. London: HMSO.

13. Personal communication with K.C. Windridge: Parenthood Research Group, University of Leicester, UK.

14. Appleby, L. (1991). Suicide during pregnancy and in the first postnatal year. *British Medical Journal*, *302* (6769), 137–40.

15. Pagel, M.D., Smilkstein, G., Regen, H. & Montano, D. (1990). Psychosocial influences on newborn outcomes: a controlled prospective study. *Social Science and Medicine*, *30* (5), 597–604.

16. Lennon, M. (1982). The psychological consequences of menopause: the importance of timing of a life stage event. *Journal of Health and Social Behaviour*, *23*, 353–66.

17. Curry, M.A. (1990). Stress, social support, and self-esteem during pregnancy. *NAACOSS Clinical Issues in Perinatal and Women's Health Nursing*, *1* (3), 303–10.

18. Cliver, S.P., Goldenberg, R.L., Cutter, G.R., Hoffman, H.J., Copper, R.L., Gotlieb, S.J. & Davis, R.O. (1992). The relationships among psychosocial profile, maternal size, and smoking in predicting fetal growth retardation. *Obstetrics and Gynecology*, *80* (2), 262–7.

19. Malley, J. & Stewart, A. (1988). Women's work and family roles: sources of stress and sources of strength. In S. Fisher & J. Reason (eds) *Handbook of Life Stress, Cognition and Health*. Chichester: John Wiley and Sons.

20. Green, J.M. (1990). 'Who is Unhappy after Childbirth?' Antenatal and intrapartum correlates from a prospective study. *Journal of Reproductive and Infant Psychology*, *8* (3), 175–83.

21. Nuckolls, K.B., Cassell, J. & Kaplan, B.H. (1972). Psychosocial assets, life crisis and prognosis of pregnancy. *American Journal of Epidemiology*, *95*, 431.

22. Lynch, J. (1977). *The Broken Heart: The Medical Consequences of Loneliness*. New York: Basic Books.

23. Collee, J. (1991). A doctor writes. *Observer* magazine (see page 66).

24. Gjerdingen, D.K., Froberg, D. & Fontaine, P. (1990). A causal model describing the relationship of postpartum health to social support, length of leave, and complications of childbirth. *Women and Health*, *16* (2), 71–87.

25. Schuman, A.N. & Marteau, T.M. (1993). Obstetricians' and midwives' contrasting perceptions of pregnancy. *Journal of Reproductive and Infant Psychology*, *11*, 115–18.

26. Berryman, J.C. & Windridge, K.C. (1991). Having a baby after 40: I. A preliminary investigation of women's experience of pregnancy. *Journal of Reproductive and Infant Psychology*, *9*, 3–18.

27. Oakley, A. (1992). Social support in pregnancy: Methodology and findings of a 1–year follow-up study. *Journal of Reproductive and Infant Psychology*, *10*, 219–31.

28. Oakley, A. (1992). Measuring the effectiveness of psychosocial interventions in pregnancy. *International Journal of Technology Assessment in Health Care*, *8*: Supplement 1, 129–38.

29. Rajan, L. & Oakley, A. (1993). No pills for heartache: the importance of social support for women who suffer pregnancy loss. *Journal of Reproductive and Infant Psychology*, *11*, 75–87.

30. Quine, L., Rutter, D.R. & Gowen, S. (1993). Women's satisfaction with the quality of the birth experience: a prospective study of social and psychological predictors. *Journal of Reproductive and Infant Psychology*, *11*, 107–13 (see page 111).

31. Thorpe, K.J., Dragonas, T. & Golding, J. (1992). The effects of psychosocial factors on the mother's emotional well-being during pregnancy: a cross-cultural study of Britain and Greece. *Journal of Reproductive and Infant Psychology*, *10*, 191–204.

32. Thorpe, K.J., Dragonas, T. & Golding, J. (1992). The effects of psychosocial factors on the mother's emotional well-being during early parenthood: a cross-cultural study of Britain and Greece. *Journal of Reproductive and Infant Psychology*, *10*, 205–17.

33. Caspar, L.M. & Hogan, D.P. (1990). Family networks in prenatal and postnatal health. *Social Biology*, *37* (1–2), 84–101.

34. *Demographic review: A report on population in Great Britain*. (1978). OPCS, Series DR, no. 1. London: HMSO.

35. *Birth Statistics, 1992*. (1994). Review of the Registrar General on births and patterns of family building in England and Wales. Series FM1, no. 21. London: HMSO.

36. Jordan, P. (1989). Support behaviours identified as helpful and desired by second-time parents over the perinatal period. *Maternal-Child Nursing Journal*, *18* (2), 133–45.

37. Linn, R. (1991). Mature unwed mothers in Israel: socio-moral and psychological dilemmas. *Lifestyles*, *12* (2), 145–70 (see page 158).

38. Wallace, P. & Gotlib, I. (1990). Marital adjustment during the tran-

sition to parenthood: stability and predictors of change. *Journal of Marriage and the Family, 52,* 21–9.

39. Englert, Y. (1994). Artificial insemination of single women and lesbian women with donor semen. *Human Reproduction, 9* (11), 1969–77.

40. Kent, A. (1989). Home is where the fear is. *Nursing Times, 85* (22), 16–17.

41. Stets, J. (1990). Verbal and physical aggression in marriage. *Journal of Marriage and the Family, 52,* 501–14.

42. Thorpe, K.J., Greenwood, R. & Little, R.E. (1994). Frequency of alcohol use, life events, and emotional status in pregnancy. University of Bristol, UK: Manuscript submitted for publication.

43. Bresnahan, K., Zuckerman, B. & Cabral, H. (1992). Psychosocial correlates of drug and heavy alcohol use among pregnant women at risk for drug use. *Obstetrics and Gynecology, 80,* 976–80.

44. Aaronson, L.S. (1989). Perceived and received support: effects on health behaviour during pregnancy. *Nursing Research, 38* (1), 4–9.

45. Berkowitz, G. & Kasl. cited in Caspar, L. M. & Hogan, D. P. (1990) op. cit.

46. Lantican, L.S.M. & Corona, D. (1992). Comparison of the social support networks of Filipino and Mexican–American primigravidas. *Health Care for Women International, 13* (4), 329–38.

47. Tomlinson, B., White, M.A. & Wilson, M.E. (1990). Family dynamics during pregnancy. *Journal of Advanced Nursing, 15,* 683–8.

48. Bowman, M. (1990). Coping efforts and marital satisfaction: measuring marital coping and its correlates. *Journal of Marriage and the Family, 52,* 463–74.

49. Belsky, J. & Rovine, M. (1990). Patterns of marital change across the transition to parenthood: pregnancy to three years postpartum. *Journal of Marriage and the Family, 52* (1), 5–20.

50. Aldous, J. (1990). Family development and the life course: two perspectives on family change. *Journal of Marriage and the Family, 52,* 571–83.

51. MacDermid, S.M., Huston, T.L. & Hale, S.M. (1990). Changes in marriage associated with the transition to parenthood: individual differences as a function of sex-role attitudes and changes in the division of household labor. *Journal of Marriage and the Family, 52,* 475–86.

52. Williams, T. et al. (1987). Transition to motherhood: a longitudinal study. *Infant Mental Health Journal, 8* (3), 251–65.

53. Lewis, J.M. (1988). The transition to parenthood: II. Stability and change in marital structure. *Family Process, 27,* 273–83.

54. Umberson, D. (1989). Relationships with children: explaining parents' psychological well-being. *Journal of Marriage and the Family, 51,* 999–1012.

8: Birth and Afterwards: Facts and Feelings

1. Shorter, E. (1984). *A History of Women's Bodies*. Middlesex: Pelican Books.
2. Berryman, J.C. & Windridge, K.C. (1994). Leicester Motherhood Project. Unpublished findings. University of Leicester, UK.
3. Kern, I. (1982). '. . . an endless joy . . .': The culture of motherhood over 35. *Papers in the Social Sciences*, 2, 43–56.
4. Heaman, M., Beaton, J., Cupton, A. & Sloan, J. (1992). A comparison of childbirth expectations in high-risk and low-risk pregnant women. *Clinical Nursing Research*, 1 (3), 252–65.
5. Quine, L., Rutter, D.R. & Gowne, S. (1993). Women's satisfaction with the quality of the birth experience: a prospective study of social and psychological predictors. *Journal of Reproductive and Infant Psychology*, 11, 107–13.
6. Nelson, M. (1982). The effect of childbirth preparation on women of different social classes. *Journal of Health and Social Behaviour*, 23, 339–52.
7. Felton, G. & Segelman, F. (1978). Lamaze Training and changes in belief about personal control. *Birth and the Family Journal*, 3 (3), 141–50.
8. Kleiverda, G., Steen, A.M., Andersen, I., Treffers, P.E. & Everaerd, W. (1991). Confinement in nulliparous women in the Netherlands: subjective experiences related to actual events and to post-partum well-being. *Journal of Reproductive and Infant Psychology*, 9, 195–213.
9. Langer, M., Czermak, B. & Ringler, M. (1990). Couple relationship, birth preparation and pregnancy outcome: a prospective controlled study. *Journal of Perinatal Medicine*, 18, 201–8.
10. Michie, S., Marteau, T.M. & Kidd, J. (1990). Antenatal Classes: Knowingly undersold. (Abstract). *Journal of Reproductive and Infant Psychology*, 8 (4), 248.
11. Gjerdingen, D., Froberg, D. & Fontaine, P. (1991). The effects of social support on women's health during pregnancy, labour and delivery, and the postpartum period. *Family Medicine*, 23 (5), 370–5.
12. Melzack, R., Taenzer, P., Feldmann, P. & Kinch, R.A. (1981). Cited in Kleiverda, G., Steen, A.M., Anderson, I., Treffers, P.E. & Everaerd, W. (1991). Confinement in nulliparous women in the Netherlands: subjective experiences related to actual events and to post-partum well-being. *Journal of Reproductive and Infant Psychology*, 9, 195–213.
13. Elliott, S. et al (1984). Relationship between obstetric outcome and psychological measures in pregnancy and the postnatal year. *Journal of Reproductive and Infant Psychology*, 2, 18–32.
14. Welles-Nystrom, B.L. & de Chateau, P. (1987). Maternal age and

transition to motherhood: prenatal and perinatal assessments. *Acta Psychiatrica Scandinavia, 76,* 719–25.

15. Younger, J. (1991). A model of parenting stress. *Research in Nursing and Health, 14,* 197–204.

16. Pridham, K.F., Lytton, D., Chang, A.S. & Rutledge, D. (1991). Early postpartum transition: progress in maternal identity and role attainment. *Research in Nursing and Health, 14,* 21–31.

17. Fridh, G. & Gaston-Johannson, F. (1990). Do primiparas and multiparas have realistic expectations of labour? *Acta Obstetrica Gynecologia Scandinavica, 69,* 103–9.

18. Green, J., Coupland, V. & Kitzinger, J. (1990). Expectations, experiences, and psychological outcomes of childbirth: a prospective study of 825 women. *Birth, 17* (1), 15–24.

19. Byrne-Lynch, A. (1990). Self-efficacy and childbirth. Paper presented as a poster at the Tenth Anniversary Conference of the Society for Reproductive and Infant Psychology. Personal communication with K.C. Windridge.

20. Byrne-Lynch, A. (1994). Psychological factors influencing medication use during childbirth. Paper presented at the Annual conference of the Society for Reproductive and Infant Psychology. 7–9 September, 1994.

21. Poore, M. & Foster, J.C. (1985). Epidural anaesthesia and no epidural anaesthesia: Differences between mothers and their experiences of birth. *Birth, 12,* 205–13. Cited in A. Byrne-Lynch (1994). op. cit.

22. Bydlowski, M. (1991). Childbirth customs: a psychoanalytical approach. *Journal of Reproductive and Infant Psychology, 9,* 35–41.

23. Klaus, M., Kennel, J., McGrath, S., Robertson, S. & Hinckley, C. (1990). The effect of social support during labor on the health of mother and infant. (Abstract). *Journal of Reproductive and Infant Psychology. 8* (4), 288.

24. Garcia, J., Kilpatrick, R. & Richards, M. (1990). *The Politics of Maternity Care: Services for Childbearing Women in Twentieth-Century Britain.* Oxford: Clarendon Press.

25. Bourne, G. (1989). *Pregnancy.* London: Pan Books Ltd.

26. Tulman, L. & Fawcett, J. (1991). Recovery from childbirth. Looking back six months after delivery. *Health Care for Women International, 12,* 341–50.

27. Gjerdingen, D.K., Froberg, D.G. & Fontaine, P. (1990). A causal model describing the relationship of women's postpartum health to social support, length of leave, and complications of childbirth. *Women and Health, 16* (2), 71–87.

28. Berryman, J.C. & Windridge, K.C. (1991). Having a baby after 40: II. A preliminary investigation of women's experience of mother-

hood. *Journal of Reproductive and Infant Psychology, 9,* 19–33.

29. MacArthur, C., Lewis, M. & Knox, E.G. (1991). *Health After Childbirth.* London: HMSO.

30. Hellin, K. & Waller, G. (1992). Mothers' mood and infant feeding: prediction of problems and practices. *Journal of Reproductive and Infant Psychology, 10* (1), 39–51.

31. Kumar, R. & Brockington, I. (eds). (1988). *Motherhood and Mental Illness. 2: Causes and Consequences.* London: Wright (see page 50).

32. York, R. (1990). Pattern of Postpartum blues. *Journal of Reproductive and Infant Psychology, 8,* 67–73.

33. Thirkettle, J.A. & Knight, R.G. (1985). The psychological precipitants of transient postpartum depression – a review. *Current Psychological Research and Reviews, 4* (2), 143–66.

34. Thune-Larsen. K.B. & Møller-Pedersen, K. (1988). Childbirth experience and postpartum emotional disturbance. *Journal of Reproductive and Infant Psychology, 6,* 229–40.

35. Dimitrovsky, L., Perez-Hirshberg, M. & Itskowitz, R. (1987). Depression during and following pregnancy: quality of family relationships. *Journal of Psychology, 121* (3), 213–18.

36. Cutrona, C.E. (1982). Nonpsychotic postpartum depression: a review of recent research. *Clinical Psychology Review, 2,* 487–503. Cited in L.C. Huffman, M. Lamour, Y.E. Bryan & F.A. Pederson (1990). Depressive symptomatology during pregnancy and the postpartum period: is the Beck Depression Inventory applicable? *Journal of Reproductive and Infant psychology, 8,* 87–97.

37. Pitt, B. (1968). 'Atypical' depression following childbirth. *British Journal of Psychiatry, 114,* 1325–35. Cited in L.C. Huffman, M. Lamour, Y.E. Bryan & F.A. Pederson (1990). Depressive symptomatology during pregnancy and the postpartum period: is the Beck Depression Inventory applicable? *Journal of Reproductive and Infant Psychology, 8,* 87–97.

38. Cox, J.L., Holden, J.M. & Sagovsky, R. (1987). Detection of postnatal depression: development of the 10–item Edinburgh Postnatal Depression Scale. *British Journal of Psychiatry, 150,* 782–6.

39. Leifer, M. (1977). Psychological changes accompanying pregnancy and motherhood. *Genetic Psychology Monographs, 95,* 55–96.

40. Thorpe, K.J., Dragonas, T. & Golding, J. (1992). The effects of psychosocial factors on the mother's emotional well-being during early parenthood: A cross-cultural study of Britain and Greece. *Journal of Reproductive and Infant Psychology, 10,* 205–17.

41. Dennerstein, L., Lehert, P. & Riphagen, F. (1989). Postpartum depression: risk factors. *Journal of Psychosomatic Obstetrics and Gynaecology Supplement, 10,* 53–65.

42. Popov, J. & Stambolova, S.V. (1990). Results from a study on frus-

tration and depression in older nulliparous women. *Akusherstve i Ginekologiia, 29* (1), 28–32.

43. Entwistle, D.R. & Goening, S.G. (1981). *The First Birth: A Family Turning Point.* Baltimore: John Hopkins University Press.
44. Price, J. (1988). *Motherhood: What it does to your mind.* London: Pandora.
45. Fisher, J.R.W., Stanley, R.O. & Burrows, G.D. (1990). Psychological adjustment to caesarean surgery: a review of the evidence. *Journal of Psychosomatic Obstetrics and Gynaecology, 11,* 91–106.
46. Thorpe, K.J., Greenwood, R. & Little, R.E. (1994). Frequency of alcohol use, life events, and emotional status in pregnancy. University of Bristol, UK: Manuscript submitted for publication.
47. Carothers, A.D. & Murray, L. (1990). Estimating psychiatric morbidity by logistic regression: Application to post-natal depression in a community sample. *Psychological Medicine, 20* (3), 695–702.
48. Brooten, D., Gennaro, S., Brown, L.P., Butts, P. et al. (1988). Anxiety, depression and hostility in mothers of preterm infants. *Nursing Research, 37* (4), 213–16.
49. Reis, J. (1988). Correlates of depression according to maternal age. *Journal of Genetic Psychology, 149* (4), 535–45.
50. Walter, C. (1986). *The Timing of Motherhood.* Lexington, Massachusetts: D.C. Heath and Company. Cited in K. Wijma & B. von Schoultz (eds). (1992). Reproductive Life: advances in research in psychosomatic obstetrics and gynaecology. The proceedings of the 10th international congress on psychosomatic obstetrics and gynaecology, held in Stockholm, Sweden, 14–17 June 1992. Carnforth, Lancashire, UK: Parthenon Publishing Group.
51. Cochran, M., Larner, M., Riley, D., Gunnarson, L. & Henderson, Jr., C.R. (1990). *Extending Families.* New York: Cambridge University Press.
52. Elliott, S. (1990). Commentary on childbirth as a life event. *Journal of Reproductive and Infant Psychology, 8,* 147–53 (see page 154).

9: Multiple Roles, Multiple Lives: Making Decisions about Paid Work

1. Behrman, D.L. (1982). *Family and/or Career: Plans of First-time Mothers.* Ann Arbor, Michigan: UNI Research Press.
2. Martin, Martin, J. & Roberts, C. (1984) *Women and Employment: A Lifetime Perspective.* London: HMSO.
3. Brannen, J. & Moss, P. (1988). *New Mothers at Work.* London: Unwin.
4. OPCS (1994). *The General Household Survey, 1991.* London: HMSO.

5. Tizard, B. (1991). Employed mothers and the care of young children. In A. Phoenix, A. Woollett & E. Lloyd (eds) *Motherhood: Meanings, Practices and Ideologies*. London: Sage.

6. Thorpe, K.J. & Cinnamon, J. (1992). The Timing of Motherhood. Unpublished research report. University of Queensland, Australia.

7. Berryman, J.C. & Windridge, K.C. (1994). Leicester Motherhood Project. Unpublished findings. University of Leicester, UK.

8. Wilkie, J.R. (1981). The trend towards delayed parenthood. *Journal of Marriage and the Family*, *43*, 583–91.

9. Olson, J.E., Frieze, I.H. & Detlefsen, E.G. (1990). Having it all? Combining work and family in a male and female profession. *Sex Roles*, *23* (9/10), 515–33.

10. Political and Economic Planning. (1971). *Women in Top Jobs*, London: Allen and Unwin.

11. Nicholson, N. & West, M.A. (1988). *Managerial Job Change: Men and Women in Transition*. Cambridge University Press.

12. Robinson, G.E., Olmstead, M., Garner, D.M. & Gare, D.J. (1989). Transition to parenthood in elderly primiparas. *Journal of Psychosomatic Obstetrics and Gynaecology*, *9*, 89–101.

13. Berryman, J.C. & Windridge, K.C. (1991). Having a baby after 40: A preliminary investigation of women's experience of pregnancy. *Journal of Reproductive and Infant Psychology*, *9*, 3–18.

14. Hoffman, L.W. & Nye, F.I. (1974). *Working Mothers*. San Francisco: Jossey-Bass.

15. Parnes, H.S., Shea, J.R., Spitz, R.S. & Zeller, F.A. (1970). *Dual Careers: A Longitudinal Study of Labor Market experience of Women*. 1, Manpower Research Monograph 21. Washing, DC: Government Printing Office.

16. Nandy, D. & Nandy, L. (1975). Towards true equality for women. *New Society*, 30 January (see page 248).

17. Oakley, A. (1974). *The Sociology of Housework*. Oxford: Martin Robertson.

18. Oakley, A. (1979). *From Here to Maternity: Becoming a Mother*. London: Penguin.

19. Oakley, A. (1980). *Women Confined: Towards a Sociology of Childbirth*. Oxford: Martin Robertson.

20. Bowlby, J. (1951). *Maternal Care and Mental Health*. Geneva: WHO.

21. Rutter, M. (1981). *Maternal Deprivation Reassessed* (2nd edition). London: Penguin.

22. Simmons, J. (1970). Why do they want to stay home? *Cornell Journal of Social Relations*, *5*, 29–39.

23. Hock, E. (1978). Working and non-working mothers with infants: Perceptions of their careers, their infants' needs, and satisfaction with mothering. *Developmental Psychology*, *14*, 37–43.

24. Birnbaum, J.A. (1975). Life patterns and self-esteem in gifted family-orientated and career-committed women. In M. Mednick, S. Tangri, and L. Hoffman (eds) *Women and Achievement*. Washington DC: Hemisphere Publishing Corporation.

25. Moss, P. (1991). Day-care for young children in the United Kingdom. In E.C. Melhuish & P. Moss (eds) *Day-care For Young Children*. London: Routledge.

26. Cooper, C.L. & Davidson, M.J. (1982). *High Pressure: Working Lives of Women Managers*. London: Fontana.

27. Scarr, S. & Dunn, J. (1987). *Mother Care, Other Care*. London: Penguin.

28. Lewis, S. (1991). Motherhood and Employment: The impact of social and organisational values. In A. Phoenix, A. Woollett & E. Lloyd (eds) *Motherhood: Meanings, Practices and Ideologies*. London: Sage.

29. Melhuish, E.C. and Moss, P. (1991). Day-care for young children in the United Kingdom. In E.C. Melhuish and P. Moss (eds) *Day-care For Young Children*. London: Routledge.

30. Gilbert, L.A. (1985). *Men in dual career families: Current realities and future prospects*. Hillsdale, N J: Erlbaum.

31. Steil, J.M. and Turetsky, B.A. (1987). Is equal better? The relationship between marital equality and psychological symptomology. *Applied Social Psychology Annual*, 7, 73–97.

32. Lewis, S. and Cooper, C.L. (1987). Stress in two-earner couples and stage in the life-cycle. *Journal of Occupational Psychology*, *60*, 289–303.

33. Scarr, S., Phillips, D. & McCartney, K. (1989). Dilemmas of child care in the United States: Working mothers and children at risk. *Canadian Psychologist*, *30*, 126–43.

34. Baruch, G., Barnett, R. & Rivers, C. (1983). *New Patterns of Love and Work for Today's Women*. New York: New American Library.

35. Crosby, F.J. (1982). *Relative Deprivation and Working Women*. New Haven: Yale University Press.

36. Malley, J.E. & Stewart, A.J. (1988). Women's work and family roles: sources of stress and sources of strength. In S. Fisher & J. Reason (eds) *Handbook of Life Stress, Cognition and Health*. Chichester: John Wiley and Son.

37. Rodin, J. & Ickovics, J.R. (1990). Women's Health: Review and research agenda as we approach the 21st century. *American Psychologist*, *45* (9), 1018–35.

38. Gjerdingen, D.K., Froberg, D.G. & Fontaine, P. (1990). A causal model describing the relationship of women's postpartum health to social support, length of leave and complications of pregnancy. *Women and Health*, *16*, (2) 71–87.

39. Hock, E. & DeMeis, D.K. (1990). Depression in mothers of infants: The role of maternal employment. *Developmental Psychology*, *26*, 285–91.

10: Older Mothers and their Children: Better Late . . . For Whom?

1. Greer, G. (1992). Women over 45 should not have babies. *Options*, November.
2. Oxford, E. (1994). Older women 'have time to make children feel important'. *Independent*, 4 January.
3. Slaughter, A. Cited in D. Danziger. (1994). My mother forced me to marry at the age of 19. *Daily Mail*, 2 June.
4. Rossan, S. (1994). Personal communication to author.
5. Price, J. (1977). *You're Not Too Old To Have a Baby*. New York: Farrar, Straus and Giroux.
6. Kern, I. (1982). '. . . an endless joy . . .': The culture of motherhood over 35. *Papers in the Social Sciences*, *2*, 43–56.
7. Ragozin, A.S., Basham, R.B., Crnic, K.A., Greenberg, M.T. & Robinson, N.M. (1982). Effects of maternal age on parenting role. *Developmental Psychology*, *18* (4), 627–34 (see page 627).
8. Mercer, R.T. (1986). *First-time Motherhood: Experiences from Teens to Forties*. New York: Springer Publishing Company (see page 35).
9. Berryman, J.C. & Windridge, K.C. (1991). Having a baby after 40. I: A preliminary investigation of women's experience of pregnancy. *Journal of Reproductive and Infant Psychology*, *9*, 3–18.
10. Berryman, J.C. & Windridge, K.C. (1991). Having a baby after 40. II: A preliminary investigation of women's experience of motherhood. *Journal of Reproductive and Infant Psychology*, *9*, 19–33.
11. Yarrow, A.L. (1991). *Latecomers – Children of Parents Over 35*. New York: The Free Press, Macmillan (see pages 104, 89, 90, 95, 104, 155, 200).
12. Berryman, J.C. & Windridge, K.C. (1992). Maternal attachment to the foetus as a function of parity and maternal age. Paper presented to the September meeting of The Society of Reproductive and Infant Psychology.
13. Thorpe, K.J. & Cinnamon, J. (1992). The Timing of Motherhood. Unpublished research report. University of Queensland, Australia.
14. Berryman, J.C. & Windridge, K.C. (1994). Leicester Motherhood Project. Unpublished findings. University of Leicester, UK.
15. McCaulay, C.S. (1976). *Pregnancy After Thirty-five*. New York: Duffon.
16. Fabe, M. & Winkler, M. (1979). *Up Against the Clock*. New York: Random House.

17. Shultz, T. (1979). *Woman Can Wait: The Pleasures of Motherhood After 30.* New York: Doubleday.
18. Rubin, S.P. (1980). *It's Not Too Late for a Baby: For Women and Men over 35.* New Jersey: Prentice-Hall.
19. Kitzinger, S. (1982). *Birth Over Thirty.* London: Sheldon Press.
20. Michelson, J. & Gee, S. (1984). *Coming Late to Motherhood.* Wellingborough: Thorsons.
21. Walter, C.A. (1984). *The Timing of Motherhood.* Lexington, Massachusetts: D.C. Heath (see pages 107, 109).
22. Bostock, Y. & Jones, M. (1987). *Now or Never? Having a Baby Later in Life.* Wellingborough: Grapevine.
23. Freely, M. & Pyper, C. (1993). *Pandora's Clock: Understanding our Fertility.* London: Heinemann.
24. Daniels, P. & Weingarten, K. (1983). *Sooner or Later: The Timing of Parenthood in Adult Lives.* New York: W.W. Norton.
25. Frankel, A. & Wise, Myra J. (1982). A view of delayed parenting: some implications of a new trend. *Psychiatry, 45* (3), 220–5.
26. Department of Health and Social Security. (1974). Present day practice in infant feeding (Reports on health and social subjects, no. 9). London: HMSO.
27. Department of Health and Social Security. (1980). Present day practice in infant feeding (Report on health and social subjects, no. 20). London: HMSO.
28. Department of Health and Social Security. (1988). Present day practice in infant feeding (Reports on health and social subjects, no. 3). London: HMSO.
29. Einon, D. (1988). *Parenthood: The Whole Story.* London: Bloomsbury.
30. Romito, P. (1988). Mothers Experience of Breastfeeding. *Journal of Reproductive and Infant Psychology. 6* (2), 89–99.
31. Berryman, J.C. & Windridge, K.C. (1994). Older Mothers: The Changing Experience of Pregnancy and Birth. *Worldview, 3* (1), 1–7.
32. Thirkettle, J.A. & Knight, R.G. (1985). The psychological precipitants of transient postpartum depression: a review. *Current Psychological Research and Reviews, 4* (2), 143–66.
33. Popov, I. & Stambolova, S. (1990). Resultati ot prouchvaneto na frustratsiiata i depresiviteta pri vuzrastni purveskini, *Akusherstve i Ginekologiia, 29* (1), 28–32.
34. Fisher, J.R.W. & Dennerstein, L. (1992). Women and the professions: when is the best time to start a family? In K. Wijma & B von Schoultz (eds) *Reproductive Life: Advances in Research in Psychosomatic Obstetrics and Gynaecology.* Lancashire: Parthenon Publishing Group.
35. Gjerdingen, D.K., Froberg, D.G. & Foutaine, P. (1990). A causal

model describing the relationship of women's postpartum health to social support, length of leave and complications of pregnancy. *Women and Health, 15* (2), 71–87.

36. Seth, M. & Khanna, M. (1978). Child rearing attitudes of the mothers as a function of age. *Child Psychiatry Quarterly, 11* (!), 6–9.

37. Sears, R.R., Maccoby, E. & Levin, H. (1957). *Patterns of Child Rearing.* Illinois: Row, Peterson and Co. (see page 436).

38. Zybert, P., Stein, Z. & Belmont, L. (1978). Maternal age and children's ability. *Perceptual and Motor Skills. 47*, 815–18.

39. Boulton, M.G. (1983). *On Being a Mother: A Study of Women with Pre-School Children.* London: Tavistock.

40. Jeffries, M. (ed) (1985). *You and Your Baby: Pregnancy to Infancy.* London: British Medical Association, Family Doctor Publication.

41. Gutman, M.A. (1985). Fertility management: Infertility, delayed childbearing and voluntary childlessness. In D.C. Goldberg (ed) *Contemporary Marriage: Special Issues in Couples Therapy.* Illinois: Dorsey Press.

42. Falbo, T. & Polit, D.F. (1986). Quantitative review of the only child literature: research evidence and theory development. *Psychological Bulletin, 100* (2), 176–89 (see page 176).

43. Falbo, T. (1987). Only children in the United States and China. *Applied Social Psychology Annual, 7*, 159–83.

44. Blum, M. (1979). Is the elderly primipara really at high risk? *Journal of Perinatal Medicine, 7*, 108–12.

45. Unpublished quote from the study published as: Berryman, J.C. (1993). Who wants egg donation? *Issue*, Winter, 13–14.

46. Dunn, J. (1982). *Sisters and Brothers.* London: Fontana.

47. Berg, I., Butler, A. & McGuire, R. (1972). Birth order and family size of school-phobic adolescents. *British Journal of Psychiatry, 121* (564), 509–14.

48. Halmi, K.A. (1974). Anorexia nervosa: demographic and clinical features in 94 cases. *Psychosomatic Medicine, 36* (1), 18–26.

49. Dalen, P. (1977). Maternal age and incidence of schizophrenia in the Republic of Ireland. *British Journal of Psychiatry, 131*, 301–5.

50. Gardner, M.J., Shee, M.P., Hall, A.J., Powell, C.A., Downes, S. & Terrell, J.D. (1990). Results of case-control study of leukaemia and lymphoma among young people near Sellafield nuclear plant in West Cumbria. *British Medical Journal, 300*, 423-34.

51. Dawson, T. Cited in L. Lee-Potter. (1994). Life without Les. *Daily Mail*, 4 May.

52. Newton, M.B. & De Issekutz-Wolsky, M. (1969). The effect on parental age of rate of female maturation. *Gerontologia, 15*, 328–31.

53. *Population Trends 75.* (1994). Spring 1994. London: HMSO.

54. *Demographic Review: a report on population in Great Britain, 1977.* (1978). Office of Population censuses and Surveys. London: HMSO.

55. *Population Trends 69.* (1992). Autumn 1992. London: HMSO.
56. Wavell, S. (1994). In the name of the father. *The Sunday Times*, 3 July.
57. Emson, H.E. (1992). A right to reproduce. *Lancet, 340*, 1083.
58. Campbell, C. Cited in Jardine, C. (1993). I had a baby at 55. *Woman*, 30 August.
59. Shaw, M. (1986). Substitute parenting. In W. Sluckin & M. Herbert (eds) *Parental Behaviour*. Oxford: Blackwell.
60. Antinori, S. Cited in J. Phillips. (1994). Woman, 62, gives birth as 'oldest mother in the world'. *The Times*, 19 July.
61. Sauer, M. (1993). In *Cheating Time*. A Horizon programme transmitted on 11 January on BBC 2. (Quotations from the published text, pages 15, 3, 11).
62. Craft, I. Cited in A. Neustatter (1993). Pioneer in the laboratory of life. *Independent*, 3 August.
63. Pallot, P. (1993). BMA chief calls for ethics guidelines. *Daily Telegraph*, 28 December.

Recommended Reading

Birke, L., Himmelweit, S. & Vines, G. (1990). *Tomorrow's Child: Reproductive Technologies in the 90's*. London: Virago. (A thought-provoking book on the advances in reproductive technology.)

Bourne, G. (1989). *Pregnancy*. London: Pan Books. (An authoritative and extremely comprehensive view of pregnancy written by an obstetrician/gynaecologist, updated in 1989. A useful source of information.)

Brannen, J. & Moss, P. (1988). *New Mothers at Work*. London: Unwin. (A very readable book giving facts and women's accounts of the experience of returning to work after having a baby.)

Byrnes, J. (1994). *Fit and Healthy at 40+*. Which Consumer Guides. London: Consumers' Association. (A helpful and readable book on keeping fit and healthy as one gets older.)

The Daycare Trust
Publications include: *ABC of Quality Childcare, Daycare for Kids, Babies in Daycare, Becoming a Breadwinner*. For details contact: The Daycare Trust, Wesley House, Wild Court, London, WC2B 4AU.

Einon, D. (1988). *Parenthood: The Whole Story*. London: Bloomsbury. (Parenthood discussed from a psychologist's viewpoint.)

Freely, M. & Piper, C. (1993). *Pandora's Clock*. London: Heinemann. (A book which helps women understand their fertility better, covering contraception, abortion, pregnancy and infertility.)

Katz Rothman, B. (1986). *The Tentative Pregnancy*. New York: Viking

Penguin. (Discusses the issues surrounding antenatal screening; particularly relevant to older mothers.)

Kitzinger, S. (1994). *The Year After Childbirth: Surviving the First Year of Motherhood*. Oxford University Press. (A realistic and reassuring book from a well-known author, covering a very wide range of issues that interest new parents of any age.)

Llewellyn-Jones, D. (1993). *Everywoman: A Gynaecological Guide for Life*. London: Penguin. (A very useful guide for all women.)

Martin, A. (1993). *The Guide to Lesbian and Gay Parenting*. London: Pandora. (A practical and ground-breaking book that discusses all the issues surrounding motherhood for lesbians.)

Mosse, K. (1993). *Becoming a Mother*. London: Virago. (This is easy to read and well-researched. It includes a section on motherhood after 35. It contains an extensive list of useful addresses for those who have experiences, or need information, not covered by most texts.)

Moulder, C. (1990). *Miscarriage: Women's Experiences and Needs*. London: Pandora. (A very useful book for any woman who has miscarried, or for those who want to help her. Its message may also be useful for partners.)

Phoenix, A., Woollett, A. & Lloyd, E. (1991). *Motherhood: Meanings, Practices and Ideologies*. London: Sage. (A range of chapters on a variety of topics of interest to mothers, including the age issue, and children with disabilities.)

Price, J. (1988). *Motherhood: What It Does to Your Mind*. London: Pandora. (An explanation of the emotional side of becoming a mother written by a psychiatrist, psychotherapist, and mother.)

Sparkes, P. (1991). *Child Care Options for the Nineties*. London: Macdonald Optima. (A book which discusses the range of options available for parents.)

Tan, S.I. & Jacobs, H.S. (1992). *Infertility: Your Questions Answered*. London: McGraw Hill. (An invaluable text for anyone wanting to know more about infertility and what can be done about it.)

Ussher, J.M. (1989). *The Psychology of the Female Body*. London: Routledge. (Looks at a range of issues and includes an excellent chapter on motherhood.)

Index